EMBRACING MY INNER ATHLETE

EMBRACING MY INNER ATHLETE

FORMER COUCH POTATO MOM DISCOVERS FITNESS, AND LIFE HASN'T BEEN THE SAME SINCE!

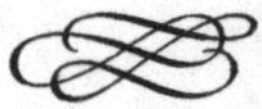

HILDEE WEISS

LIBRARY TALES PUBLISHING

Published by Library Tales Publishing
www.LibraryTalesPublishing.com

This book is a work of creative nonfiction. Some names and identifying details have been changed to protect the privacy of individuals.

9798894410326

Library Tales Publishing supports the right to free expression and the value of diverse voices. The views expressed in this work are those of the author.

CONTENTS

"Running is the best metaphor for life I know. One's running journey often includes highs and lows, good times and bad, exhilarating growth and frustrating stagnation, and unexpected twists and turns. It sounds a lot like life to me.

In *Embracing My Inner Athlete,* Hildee Weiss details her journey from "couch potato mom" to accomplished runner, and all of the highlights and lowlights she has experienced along the way. Hildee also includes many stories from her personal life in this book, and it's not surprising to note that her running and her life often follow parallel tracks of ups and downs.

One aspect of Hildee's journey that is very apparent is that running has changed and evolved for her, rather significantly, over the years. As she has grown and changed as a human, woman, wife, mother, grandmother, and friend, the role running plays in her life has changed along with her.

Running has been a solo endeavor at times, but it also has been a way for her to connect socially with others. It's been a chance to connect and deepen friendships but also something she's been able to enjoy with various members of her family.

Running has been a central tenet of her health and fitness regimen, but she's also pulled back from running at times to focus on building strength or participate in other forms of cardio like swimming. She's run races of both longer and shorter distances and challenged herself to step outside of her comfort zone with races on trails and through mud while navigating various obstacles.

While running hasn't always looked the same for Hildee throughout her journey, it has been a vital component of her life that has helped her to become the woman she is today. Her running journey will continue to change and evolve as she progresses through life well into the future, just like it has since she took her first steps in 2014.

Hildee's story, which she shares so honestly in the pages that follow, is one that all of us can and will relate to in one way or another. Because Hildee's story is ultimately a human story, the story of a woman who has had various struggles in the past and who continues to have various struggles in her future, but does her best every day to overcome her current struggles to be the best version of Hildee Weiss that she can be.

I attempt to do the same thing every day, and I know that you do, too.

As you read through this book, I have no doubt that you'll be inspired by Hildee and the path she has traveled to this point. I also have no doubt that Hildee's story will make you wonder about your future and the possibilities that await you when you say yes to opportunities in the future, even when the opportunity scares you a little bit."

—Denny Krahe

Host of *Diz Runs Podcast*

Author of *Be Ready on Race Day: How to Create a Custom Training Plan for Your Next Marathon or Half Marathon*

❋

"I thoroughly enjoyed reading Hildee's new book, *Embracing My Inner Athlete*. Her story is a powerful, heartfelt testament to the transformative power of running. In sharing her deeply personal journey—full of triumphs, setbacks, growth, and resilience—Hildee brings a voice that is both refreshingly authentic and incredibly inspiring.

Hildee doesn't sugarcoat the struggles, and that's exactly what makes her journey so powerful. I've been grateful to get to know Hildee on a personal level, and I love how we both understand running is much more than just the miles—it's the mindset, the hard days, and the breakthroughs.

This book captures that spirit beautifully. It's more than a running memoir; it's a reminder that it's never too late to start something new, to take ownership of your health, and to discover strength you didn't know you had.

Hildee shows us what's possible when you show up for yourself with consistency, dedication, and heart. She writes with honesty, humor, and wisdom, offering not just inspiration but a practical path for others to follow. Whether you're a seasoned runner or just thinking about lacing up your shoes for the first time, her story will move you—and motivate you.

This manuscript is a gift to the running community and to anyone looking for the courage to begin something new.

Truly honored to call you a friend."

—Beatie Deutsch
Israeli National Marathon Champion

❄

CHAPTER 1

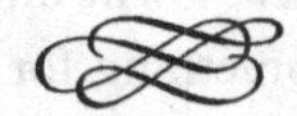

YOU'VE GOT THIS

It was Saturday, June 7, 2014, and I had just left my house to walk the three blocks to our synagogue to hear my son chant the Torah reading. As I walked along the sidewalk, I tripped on some uneven pavement, and down I went.

As I typically do to stop a fall or make it any worse than it has to be (I am not new to tripping!), I used my right hand to break my fall. I landed on my right side, hitting the ground with my right shoulder and scraping my right knee in the process. My pantyhose were torn, my knee was bleeding, and I hurt everywhere, but somehow I managed to get back on my feet and walk home, only half a block away.

I was so worried that I had broken my shoulder or kneecap that I didn't think about any damage I had done to my right hand. I could see my ring and pinky fingers swelling and looking pretty claw-like, so I removed my wedding ring and thought nothing more of it.

After the Sabbath, I went to the emergency room, where they diagnosed me with a contusion on my knee, a sore shoulder, and soft tissue damage in my hand. I was given instructions to go for occupational therapy to help with my hand injury, and that was that.

Well, not really. I scheduled my hand therapy to start in July, and in the meantime, Advil and Tylenol became my friends. My in-laws took my husband and me on a week-long cruise to the Mediterranean for our 25th anniversary, and I didn't give much thought to my hand injury.

While on the cruise, I had a one-on-one talk with my father-in-law, who expressed concern about my well-being. He recognized that I had so much going on as a wife and mother, and he wanted to ensure that I was doing something for myself. I shared with him that I had been thinking about joining the local Jewish Community Center and hiring a personal trainer or taking some classes once we returned home.

Upon returning home, I called the director of the fitness center and explained that I wanted to start working with a personal trainer but had a hand injury to consider. He suggested that I meet a trainer named Jeff for a free jumpstart session, as he was known to not only be a superb trainer but also great at working around injuries and other health restrictions.

I met Jeff one July morning at the JCC, and we went over what I had been doing for exercise. I shared with him how I did indoor walking DVDs a few mornings a week, walking anywhere between four and seven miles a day. He asked what I had been doing for resistance/weight training, and I proudly told him that I was a regular Firm workout gal, using three or five-pound weights in the cardio/toning workouts. He noted that while that was all well and good, neither the walking nor the Firm workouts were doing much for my heart rate.

We discussed my hand injury, and he assured me we would work around it and still make the most of our 30-minute sessions. Jeff then asked me to tell him the one thing I wished I could do, fitness-wise… a goal, perhaps. I told him that I wished I could run or jog, but I really didn't think I could do either.

I can't remember if I actually confided in him about my fears of how I would look in running clothes and how worried I was about my appearance while running (cue Phoebe running through Central Park in that infamous *Friends* episode). I was scared that I would trip and fall and wind up hurting myself, and of course, there was that fear of how running (if I ever actually went out and did it!) would damage my knees. Conversation over, I never gave it a second thought.

Well, Jeff apparently remembered our conversation because once my hand injury was healed and I was able to transition to one-hour workout sessions on Tuesday and Thursday mornings, I somehow found myself running on a treadmill. As a complement to our workouts, Jeff had me do intervals on the treadmill where I walked for a few minutes and then jogged for a minute. The jog soon turned into a run—not all that fast, but something that increased my heart rate.

Before I knew it, it was April of 2015, and every now and then, Jeff would mention my doing a 5K, but I said absolutely not. I had never run for more than a minute or two, and that was pretty far off from running a 5K.

One day after we had finished training, he had me go on the treadmill and set it up for me to run a mile. It's all such a blur now, but I did it, undoubtedly with a look of wonder and shock on my face (and the emergency safety clip holding me tight!) as I plodded along. A week or so later, I was back on the treadmill, but this time, I was set up to run a 5K.

I was so unsure that I could really do it, but off I went, with that emergency safety clip clipped tight to my shirt. I have no recollection of the time it took or what my pace was—ironic since I would soon become obsessed with those numbers. I do know that while I was running, I felt like I was having an out-of-body experience, and at no time did I worry about what I looked like in my outfit or how silly I might have appeared moving around on the run.

When the run was completed, I half-heartedly registered for the Beechbrook 5K with a promise from Jeff that he would be there with me on race day.

A week or so later, Jeff and I met up at the JCC after he had finished work for the day, and we headed outside for a pre-race prep 5K run around the area. I was so new to all of this that I didn't think about how we would track the run, but Jeff had it all worked out. He had this app on his watch called *Runkeeper*, and every five minutes, a voice told us our pace and what our distance was so far.

I'm sure I was huffing and puffing along the way as I felt out of shape, tired, and depleted of energy... but I also felt a sense of excitement over having run the 5K distance in 35 minutes. I had no idea that day that I would be downloading that Runkeeper app to use as a tracker for all my future exercise activities, and I had no clue at all that I would soon be going beyond the 5K distance.

That moment I signed up for that 5K was the beginning of a journey that has seen me go from sedentary wife and mother of five to a fifty-something quasi-athlete. I still have a hard time calling myself an athlete.

I was so excited and nervous when I went to pick up my race packet at the local sporting goods store that was sponsoring the race. I gave them my name, and upon receiving my t-shirt and bib, I was told to take safety pins for pinning the bib. I had all kinds of questions...

Do I need to take more than four?

Do I pin the bib to the front of my shirt or the back?

If I choose to pin it to the front, do I pin it all the way on top or towards the bottom of my shirt?

And wait... I'm not sure what I am going to wear.

Do I go ahead and wear the shirt they gave me in the race packet, or do I wear my own shirt?

So many questions...

May 10 approached, and I drove myself to the shopping center where the starting line was in the middle of the parking lot. Gary had something going on that morning, so he came to meet me to wish me luck but then had to leave. My good friend, Dina, had also signed up for the 5K, so it was great to see her there.

Jeff arrived a few minutes before the race with his wife, Mirvat, and told me he would be running the race with her but had total faith that I could do this. Hearing this, I wasn't so sure I could. I didn't know where I was going from one step to the next, but Dina and Jeff each assured me that there would be signs along the way and I should just follow the people in front of me. And so I did.

I crossed the starting line and set off on the course, exiting the parking lot and going across the street to navigate the roads surrounding a school, then looping back towards the parking lot where the finish line stood. I remember starting out, feeling a sense of being alone, yet there were a few hundred people running this with me, so I really wasn't alone.

And I certainly didn't finish alone, as Dina met me at the mile 3 mark, having already completed her own race. She cheered me on, telling me, "You've got this," and ran alongside me until I reached the finish line. Every time I recall that race, I get choked up and think about what a gift that was. She gave me that boost of confidence and assurance that I wasn't alone and that she had my back.

I finished in 30:54… a 9:56 minute mile overall pace. Not bad for a first timer!

CHAPTER 2

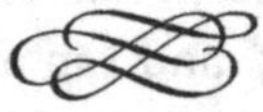

FALL. HEAL. RISE. RUN

I wasn't done running on that fateful Sunday morning in May; if anything, it marked the beginning of my journey into racing. I started running a few times a week through my neighborhood, gaining endurance and increasing my pace.

Four weeks after the Beechbrook 5K, I participated in the Gathering Place Race for the Place 5K. The Gathering Place supports cancer patients, survivors, and their families, so this 5K resonated with me. I have lost too many relatives and friends to cancer, so the race entry fee felt meaningful—a tribute to each of them.

I felt the same nervousness when picking up my race packet and again on race day. The race starts on a road just outside our local mall, winds through our neighborhood, and returns to the mall parking lot, making the route very familiar. As I ran along one street, I saw several friends and neighbors outside their homes, cheering us on. I waved as I passed them, appreciating their heartfelt support. I finished the race in 28:07, achieving a 9:03 minute mile pace overall. I had come a long way in just four weeks.

My training sessions with Jeff had increased in intensity. He introduced me to burpees, jump squats, planks, and lunges. When I wasn't running, I used the elliptical, which was a great calorie burner and effectively worked my glutes and legs.

With my hand injury behind me, I used 10-pound weights for bicep curls, tricep extensions, chest flies, and overhead presses. Jeff created workout plans for me to follow while I was out of town, as taking a break was never an option.

In the early days of building my strength and mobility, I needed a lot of guidance regarding weights and repetitions, but the exercises soon became familiar and easy. During these sessions, in between sets, Jeff and I would chat about everything under the sun—his running, my kids. He was and always would be my trainer, but he also became a dear friend in the process.

I continued running over the next several weeks, and all my initial fears about how I looked in my running clothes or how I moved faded away. Jeff talked about expanding my running horizons and training for the 10K distance, but I didn't think much of it. Maybe I heard him, but I didn't believe I had it in me to pursue such a goal.

It wasn't until August 19, when we were driving separately to meet for a mile repeat run at Acacia Reservation, that we discussed finding a 10K race. The park is just a few minutes' drive from my house, as is the JCC, so we planned to run right after Jeff finished work.

A mile repeat run consists of running one mile at a challenging pace with a short recovery in between repetitions. In our case, we would warm up with a few minutes of walking, then run a mile at eight minutes and fifty seconds, three times, with a two or three-minute walk in between.

The first mile went well, and we completed it in nine minutes and two seconds. After walking a few minutes to recover, we began the second mile, finishing it in eight minutes and forty-six seconds. Great—only one more mile to go, but I really needed to use the bathroom.

I told Jeff I needed a potty break, and he suggested I wait until we finished the third mile repeat, but I really had to go. I promised him I would be quick and hurried off.

A minute later, as I exited the restroom eager to return to our run, I tripped on the step leading from the restroom to the path. I fell hard, but after a moment, I stood up and started walking toward Jeff.

As I walked, I felt immense pain in my right foot, and my walking quickly turned into a hobble. I was close to tears, realizing the rest of the run was over. Jeff walked me to my car, assuring me I would be okay and suggesting I go home to ice and elevate my foot.

After nearly an hour of keeping my foot elevated on my old pregnancy pillow with no relief, I knew I had done something serious. My ankle was swelling, and I suspected I had sprained or possibly broken it.

I called my husband at work, and he suggested I call a friend to take me to the emergency room, where he would meet us. The X-rays didn't show any fractures, but since I was in terrible pain, I was given crutches to use "as long as it hurt."

The pain persisted for another ten days, leading me to visit our podiatrist for a second opinion. He took X-rays of my entire foot and informed me that my ankle wasn't the issue—I had broken my fifth metatarsal in the fall and needed to stay off my foot for six weeks while wearing a boot.

Six weeks—my mind raced with possibilities. I couldn't do any weight-bearing activities, meaning no running, walking, or elliptical. What could I do? What would happen to my weight if I couldn't engage in "real" exercise? Would I ever run again?

Not being able to run or walk for six weeks felt like torture. It's ironic that I spent the first forty-something years of my life avoiding physical activity, and after just a few months of running and getting good at it, it was taken away from me. I *felt* it was taken from me—yet I was the one who made that choice when I stopped my run with Jeff to go to the bathroom.

Would I have tripped on that step if I had completed the three miles without rushing? I will never know, and I can't go back in time, but I mentally berated myself for that decision countless times.

I could still exercise during those six weeks, just not at the intensity I had achieved. Jeff proved to be as great as the JCC fitness director had promised. Since I couldn't do any weight-bearing activities, I was limited to the recumbent bike for cardio—no elliptical, no arc trainer, no walking or running.

Jeff suggested I turn the pedal around on the recumbent bike so I could rest my fancy boot on it while working out on non-training days. During our training sessions, he had me off my right foot while still allowing me to work on my strength.

By mid-October, he introduced me to the TRX, a suspension training device that uses body weight for strength and conditioning. Once the six weeks were over and my doctor cleared me for weight-bearing activities, I was eager to try running again.

Not so fast, Jeff warned.

He devised a plan where I walked five minutes on the treadmill a few times a week for the first week, then added five minutes each week for three weeks. Then, I started running—five minutes the first week, adding another five each week for three more weeks.

I had stopped running on August 19 and didn't officially return until early December. But when I tied my shoelaces for my first 'real' run of more than 20 minutes, I was pain-free and fully healed.

Being sidelined for those months felt torturous, but I learned the hard way that patience is a virtue—and my recovery couldn't be rushed.

That first 'real' run was in Central Park during a long weekend in New York City. The year before, I had begun to embrace the idea of running and fantasized about returning to Central Park.

While dating Gary, I enjoyed a brief walk with him through the park and felt wistful watching others run or jog along the paths. I wished I could be one of them, but I couldn't imagine it.

Fast forward to years later—two 5K races under my belt, back to running after being sidelined for three months—I was determined to run in Central Park.

So, I did.

I turned on my Runkeeper app, and off I went. It felt so good and freeing to run along the park's pavement. I ran toward the Central Park Zoo, then turned around to return to the entrance and hit stop.

I was eager to see how far I'd gone and my pace, but somehow I had hit the elliptical button instead of the run button, so the stats were all messed up. I thought I would never know what that run truly meant.

But I did discover its significance.

It wasn't about how fast I ran or how quickly I finished; it was about turning a dream into reality and returning to something I had come to love.

In January 2016, I began running beyond four miles and started training for my first 10K. I signed up for the Cleveland Rite Aid Marathon 10K, feeling somewhat dazed but excited nonetheless.

By early February, my four-mile runs had turned into five miles, and by late February, I completed a six-mile run on the treadmill in fifty-four minutes and fifty-nine seconds. I was back at it—my paces were improving, and I felt strong.

I even tackled a few seven-plus mile runs, unsure why I needed to exceed the 6.25-mile distance of a 10K, but I discovered I was capable of it.

My workouts with Jeff increased in intensity, matching my running progress. I learned to conquer walking push-ups, Bulgarian lunges, and single-leg deadlifts. Deadlifts were the one exercise I needed to improve, and it would take years and a lot of patience to master the proper form.

May 15 arrived, and it was race day. I felt nervous and anxious, using the porta potty more times than I could count before the race began. I lined up with thousands of runners in my assigned corral, and when the gun went off, I was off.

I tracked my run on Runkeeper (making sure it was set to run and not elliptical!) and followed the arrows and signs to the finish. Runkeeper recorded my finish time as 56:05, while the official race clock showed 57:09. Honestly, I didn't care about that extra minute. I finished 394th out of 1,954 overall, with a 9:11 minute mile pace.

This was just a year after my first 5K and 13 months after I first laced up my sneakers to run. Gary was there at the finish to give me a hug and take me home, where I rode an emotional high for a day or two.

The following month, I ran my fastest 5K at the Gathering Place Race for the Place. It was the same course as the previous year, and I somehow shaved off more than a minute with a finish time of 26:48.

My training sessions with Jeff became more intense, and he frequently suggested that I consider a half marathon. Each time he brought it up, I would respond with a firm *"no way,"* much like I had when he mentioned the 10K before the one I ran in May. The thought of running twice the distance of a 10K made me think again with a resolute *"no way, no how."*

I didn't believe I could run 13.1 miles, nor could I envision following a training plan for it. Granted, I had managed to prepare for the 10K by following a plan Jeff created for me, but a 10K felt achievable. Then I remembered the previous summer when I had also said *"no way"* to Jeff about running a 10K. If a 10K turned out to be not only doable but successful, couldn't a half marathon be similarly attainable?

In what felt like another out-of-body experience, I signed up for the River Run Half Marathon scheduled for September 11. Jeff promised to run this race with me and assured me he would create a plan to prepare me for race day. He warned me that I would lose weight with all the training we would do together, along with the running I would do on my own.

I did indeed lose weight, reaching a level I hadn't seen since I was 16! I had no issue with that whatsoever!

Half marathon training officially started in mid-June with an eight-mile run on the treadmill as a baseline. The plan called for me to run four times a week, with my long run on Fridays and a mix of speed intervals, timed runs, and easy runs.

I ran outside as often as possible for my long runs to experience the full effects of road running versus treadmill running. I was doing all of this in the humid summer months, and it wasn't until late August that I felt the repercussions of running in the heat.

I met Jeff at the Rocky River Reservation for an eight-mile long run since it was part of the half marathon course, providing a great opportunity to practice on the roads. My splits for that run were all in the ten to ten-forty minute range, and I felt fine throughout — or so I thought.

When Jeff's father picked us up from the other end of the metro park, I noticed a metallic taste in my mouth. I didn't know what to make of it, but Jeff assured me it was just a bit of heat exhaustion. I couldn't recall experiencing that during my previous outdoor runs, so I chalked it up to a one-time occurrence.

Each week, I added half a mile to my long run distance, and before I knew it, I had completed a twelve-mile run without stopping in under two hours! I was ready for this half marathon.

My mind was ready... my body was ready... everything was in line when I met Jeff at the starting line of the River Run half. Gary was there as my driver, cheerleader, and photographer. He took some great pictures of me standing at the starting line.

As they played the National Anthem that day, September 11, I reflected on how our world had changed fifteen years ago with the 9/11 attacks. The song was sung with so much emotion, and it felt strange to shift from somber to excited as we prepared for the gun to go off. I also thought about how just a year ago, I was in a boot and unable to run, and the year before that, running wasn't even in my vocabulary.

Then off we went, crossing the starting line and beginning a 13.1-mile journey to the finish. Jeff and I chatted along the way, which helped distract me from checking my watch for our time and pace. The run felt manageable; the first four miles were all in the nines, and the remaining miles were in the ten to ten-and-a-half range, so I was doing well for my first half marathon.

The race was mostly flat, as promised, but there were some rolling hills around mile 9, which Jeff had warned me about. He kept encouraging me, telling me, "You've got this," which helped as we tackled mile 10, mile 11, and mile 12. With just a mile and a tenth left, I knew I truly had it. As we completed mile 13, I could see the finish line ahead and ran toward it with excitement.

We finished the race together in 2:15:40, and I felt absolutely glorious—on top of the world.

I wasn't done with just one half marathon, as I barely had time to recover from the River Run before Jeff asked me what I would do next. Races were mostly over by the time I returned in the fall of 2016 from spending a few weeks in Israel, where my husband and I were building an apartment.

We had begun spending more time in Israel since some of our children had moved there after high school for army/national service and later to attend university. We had started traveling to Israel more regularly over the past year and decided to get our own place instead of staying at someone's house or a hotel.

I tried to find a race or two in November and December when I knew I would be back in Cleveland, but I didn't find anything worthwhile. I became somewhat of a regular in the Friday morning spin classes at the J, but once winter came, I spent more time on the treadmill and elliptical than on the spin bike.

CHAPTER 3

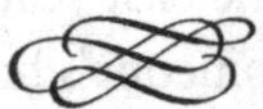

THE DAY MY LEGS GAVE OUT

In the early months of 2017, I worked out and participated in all my activities indoors at the JCC. I used the elliptical and ran and walked on the treadmill during the cold Cleveland winter. My pace improved as I did longer runs, and I found myself signing up for the Cleveland Rite Aid Half Marathon in May. Once again, Jeff would be my running partner, and this time, we aimed for a two-hour finish.

I started with a four-mile run in late February and increased the distance by a mile each week. Mile repeats and speed intervals were my go-to workouts for improving my pace, while long runs helped build my endurance. The training for this half was harder than for my first, and Jeff had warned me it would be. He cautioned that training for the second half would be a completely different experience than my River Run training, and he was right. I hadn't paid much attention when he said that, but I realized the second time around isn't as much fun.

I found I didn't enjoy the long runs this time and lacked the fresh, carefree outlook I had felt just six or seven months before. Since most of the training took place in February, March, and April, I opted to do my long runs on the treadmill instead of outside. When I did run outside, I often stopped midway because I felt too tired and had to switch to walking, ultimately cutting the run short. I felt something was wrong since I had completed the same long runs seamlessly the first time.

Jeff repeated his warning after I shared that a nine-mile long run had gone downhill—and I wasn't referring to the elevation. On the treadmill, I was fine; my paces ranged from nine to nine-forty minutes, and I never felt the need to take a break as I did outside. That April, I met Jeff for a run at Rocky River Reservation, the same metropark where I had run my first half. We hadn't run together since the River Run half, and it was great to be somewhere other than the treadmill. I didn't even think of stopping when the run felt challenging. I gave it my all, even though my paces slowed with each mile.

April turned into May, and race day was approaching. I tapered the week before the race, running three to five-mile distances at most and not pushing too hard on pace. I was ready for this race, as tough as the training had been.

A few days before the race, my friend Frankie picked up my race packet since the pick-up location was downtown, close to the courthouse where she works as a judge. She reviewed the race course map and told me that the first few miles were smooth, followed by a steep downhill at the Flats, which then led to a challenging uphill. I realized I had never consciously considered hills or felt afraid of them...until that moment.

That Friday afternoon, I called Jeff and shared my concerns, and he assured me that we would be fine and that I was ready for this.

It was May 21, race day. Gary drove me downtown with our 17-year-old son and his two friends. The three boys (now 25 but still 'boys' to me) had decided two or three weeks before the race that they wanted to run the 10K portion. None had ever participated in a race before, nor had they run a 10K distance. I had told my son, Yonatan, to do a run or two on the treadmill in our bedroom for practice. Ironically, each of the three boys placed in the top ten of their age group for the 10K, and one of them took up track running and became a bit of a running superstar!

As for me, I lined up at the starting line with Jeff at my side, feeling nervous. I had a two-hour finish time in my head but wasn't sure how it would work out, considering the weather was in the lower 70s and quite humid. I calculated that we needed to average a 9:07–9:12 minute mile. My training runs had been steady in the nine to ten-minute range, and I knew you run faster in a race due to the adrenaline.

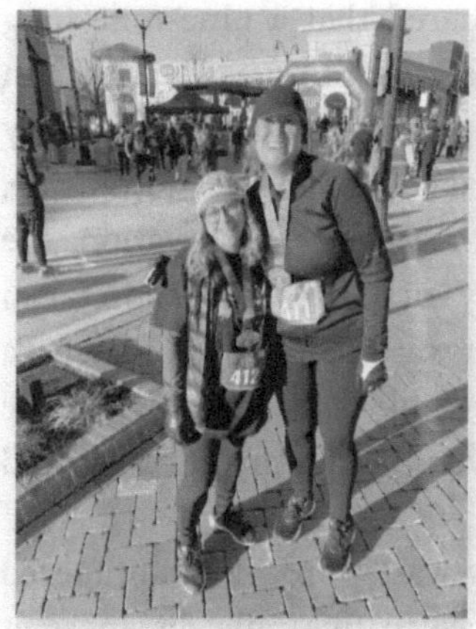

© 2020 Harry Newmark

I thought of that two-hour goal as we joined the crowd at the starting line, and off we went. Jeff tracked our pace on his watch while I monitored my own. Our first two miles were in the higher eight-minute range, and the third and fourth miles were in the lower nine-minute range. We were doing well with our pace, so I was puzzled when Jeff told me to slow down a bit.

Mile 5 had us at a 10:25 minute mile pace, and we ran a 9:54 minute mile pace for mile 6. We ran miles 7 through 13 in the 10:01–10:44 minute mile range, but I felt myself slowing as the humidity and temperature rose. I saw on my watch that we reached an hour and fifty-eight minutes at mile 12, so we weren't going to meet that two-hour finish time, but we were only a mile and a tenth from the finish line.

As we approached the bridge leading to the street where the finish line stood, I suddenly lost all feeling in my legs. My legs buckled, and I went down as carefully as I could without falling. I started to panic and cry as Jeff crouched beside me, telling me to take a moment before getting back up.

A member of the medical team approached and asked if I was okay. I assured her I was fine and would try to get up in a minute. When I attempted to stand, I quickly went back down; I couldn't support myself. I couldn't believe I was less than a quarter mile from the finish and unable to move. Runners passed by, and I felt defeated. How would I ever get up and reach the finish line? I hadn't stopped my watch—I had forgotten to press 'stop,' so the time was ticking away.

After about fifteen or sixteen minutes on the ground, I somehow managed to get up and started walking/hobbling toward the finish line. Jeff offered encouraging words, telling me how great I was and that it was just heat exhaustion. I think I was in such a bad headspace that I couldn't absorb what he was saying.

We crossed the finish line together in 2:23:32. While I turned off my watch, I kept going to meet Gary and told him I just wanted to get home. He said he had been worried about me, as he had been tracking my race and couldn't understand what had happened around mile 13 when the tracker suddenly stopped. I explained that I had gone down but hadn't hurt myself. I felt defeated, disappointed, and frustrated with myself. I had put so much work into training for this race, and this wasn't how it was supposed to go.

My oldest daughter got married on June 18, and I wore the dress of my dreams as the mother of the bride. It was a fitted navy gown with a bow on one shoulder, and I felt regal and slim. Of course, I did a run that morning, but I kept it inside and wore my emergency strap to stay upright!

The intensity of my workouts increased over the months. Jeff had me flipping a tire repeatedly across the personal training room. I started with a 95-pound tire but soon progressed to flipping a 125-pound tire—completely unaware of the benefits this movement was providing!

In early June, I reached my lowest weight of 166 pounds, but I would soon see it rise to the mid-170s for the rest of the year.

In mid-October, I took Jeff's suggestion to add swimming as a form of exercise. I wasn't bored with my running—my paces remained strong and steady—but I was open to new challenges. Swimming, however, was completely outside my comfort zone.

First of all, I hadn't worn a bathing suit in public since my teenage years. And second, I hadn't entered a swimming pool unless I was rescuing one of my kids! The first time I got into the water at the JCC pool, Jeff stood on the sidelines and instructed me on how to do a breaststroke. It had been three decades since I last swam laps, but by the end of that introductory swim class, it all started coming back to me.

Initially, I was anxious about walking out of the women's shower room in a bathing suit, but I soon realized no one was looking! Over the next several months, I committed to one day a week in the indoor pool, gradually increasing my lap count and genuinely enjoying my time in the water. Swimming was a completely different kind of workout from running, the elliptical, and spinning—but I enjoyed them all nonetheless.

While running outside in Jerusalem, I decided to sign up for the Jerusalem Marathon 10K. It was scheduled for March 2018, and I already knew the hills would be brutal. I didn't really want to do it, but I felt compelled—my kids had raved about the race for years. I'd heard it could get very humid, and I still carried a touch of PTSD from my Rite Aid Half Marathon, when I collapsed from heat exhaustion. I was also nervous about the crowds. I had a long list of reasons not to sign up… but even more reasons to go for it.

Our close friends promised to run the 10K with me, and my husband and two kids signed up as well. With that kind of support, I realized I had no reason to be afraid. I posted my intentions on Instagram, still uncertain about my decision, but a few friends commented that I looked happy and fit. Happy, yes—I was loving my time in Israel with my family. Fit, though? That word was harder. "Fit" was a compliment I struggled to accept. It didn't feel like it belonged to me… at least not yet.

CHAPTER 4

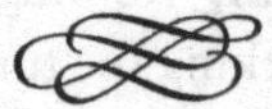

THE GIRL WHO RAN ANYWAY

The beginning of 2018 found me featured in a major ad campaign for the JCC called *"What Is Your 2018 Going to Look Like?"* A few months earlier, a marketing staffer at the J had asked Jeff to discuss sharing my story as a late-in-life runner and fitness enthusiast.

When Jeff forwarded her email to me, kindly urging me to participate, I felt conflicted. On one hand, I was uncomfortable being the center of attention and appearing in various ads and marketing materials. On the other hand, I wanted to support Jeff, an amazing trainer, and I believed this campaign would benefit the JCC in many ways.

In the end, the latter won out—although if you catch the video where I share my story, you can clearly see my discomfort in front of the camera. In the video, I explained how I joined the JCC at 45 and demonstrated that it's never too late to start being active. I also mentioned that thanks to Jeff's coaching, I feel and look better at 49 than I did at 29 and 39.

The ad campaign seemed successful; at least a few people approached me over the next few months, telling me how inspired they were by my story.

My weight stayed in the mid to high 170s for the first half of

2018, but one day I saw 181 on the scale. As someone who weighed herself every day except for my Jewish Sabbath, I freaked out when I saw that number. I worried that 181 would continue to rise and ultimately reach my starting Weight Watchers weight of 198.

Seeing that 181 marked the beginning of my obsession with the scale. I began to view that number as a measure of my success or failure, allowing it to dictate whether I was doing a 'good job' or a 'bad job.' I started to see my running and cardio workouts as a means to burn calories, marking the turning point where I began to view exercise as something I *had* to do rather than something I *wanted* to do.

In early January, I began training for the Jerusalem Marathon 10K. I returned to mile repeats, speed intervals, and hill intervals to prepare for the hills my middle daughter, Miriam, had warned me about.

I spent eight weeks training for the 10K, focusing on conditioning myself for the hills while trying not to obsess over the weather on race day. Without consulting Jeff, I did hill interval runs each week on the treadmill, gradually increasing the incline. I was doing incline bursts at 5%, 6%, and 7%, feeling completely fine.

I was determined and motivated to be ready for this 10K, hills and all. I completed most of my runs at the JCC but also trained while in Florida for winter break with our two younger kids.

Gary and I flew to Israel the week before the race and spent time with our two older kids living there. Seth was attending university after serving in the Israeli Defense Forces, and Miriam was doing her year of national service at a Jerusalem hospital.

Before I knew it, it was Friday morning, March 9, and I was standing on the grounds of Gan Sacher/Sacher Field for my first destination race. We were staying at a hotel since we didn't have our own place at the time, and Gary's brother was picking us up before 6 AM to head to the race.

Although the 10K wouldn't start until a few hours after Seth and Gary began their races (the full marathon and the 5K, respectively), I was fine with getting up early and going with Gary's brother as our driver. With many roads in Jerusalem closed for the race, Zev navigated us through the detours to reach the race location.

As we waited for our races to start, we had a chance to explore the grounds of Gan Sacher, visit the various sponsor tents, and catch up with friends who had come from all over Israel to participate. We said goodbye to Seth at 7 and wished Gary well at 7:30, leaving us two hours to hang out.

Miriam and I met up with our friends Lisa and Joel and their kids and planned to start the 10K together. Lisa and I had discussed for weeks our goal to finish in under an hour and twenty minutes, while Miriam would run her own race.

We lined up at the start at 9:15 with 20,000 people around us, all excited to race. The gun went off at 9:30, and we were off.

I stayed close to Lisa and her family for the first two kilometers, which included running up a steep street leading to downtown Jerusalem. Once we reached the top, we separated, and I moved ahead along Jaffa Street, pleasantly surprised by the many people—policemen, Israeli Defense Force soldiers, spectators—cheering us on.

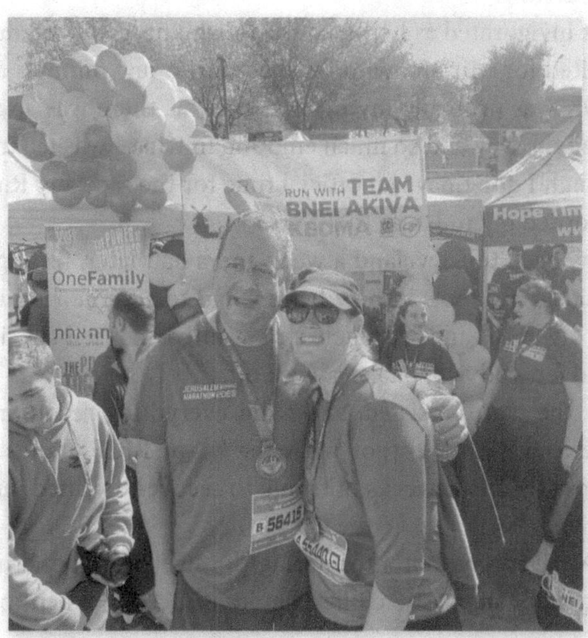

© 2018 Miriam Weiss

I especially loved running through the gates of the Old City and down a ramp, where I heard someone calling after me. It was Miriam, and we exchanged high fives before going our separate ways down the hill outside the Old City.

Ahead was a big hill, and I trotted up to the top when I noticed my Runkeeper had stopped around the four-mile mark. I took a few seconds to catch my breath and restart the app, disappointed that I wouldn't have complete tracking of the race.

I made my way around the First Station and up the street that turns onto Jabotinsky Street—THE street. Miriam had warned me that this street was steep and relentless, and she was right!

I finally reached the top and turned onto a street that took me through Rechavia. As I ran along Aza Street and passed my late great-grandfather's house at number 24 Aza, I said to myself a little too loudly, "Look at me now."

I reflected on how inactive and unhealthy I had been when I last passed his house 33 years ago, feeling proud that I was now completing this 10K. As I exited Aza and turned onto Rupin Street, which leads to the finish line, I channeled my inner runner and finished strong.

I felt invigorated as I crossed the finish line, collected my medal, and waited for Miriam, who finished only a few minutes after me. This 10K was probably my favorite race, as there was so much to see along the way and so much emotion in what I was feeling.

Though I don't have an official time for the race, my Runkeeper app recorded my finish at 1:07:56.

I flew back to Cleveland a week and a half later, feeling significant pain in my foot. I knew better than to resume running right after a big race, and as much as I wanted to get back into it, I followed Jeff's advice to take a week off.

Still, the pain persisted, and I did everything recommended—rest, ice, elevation. I forgot what the 'C' in RICE stands for, but after more than two weeks of trying to recover, I visited our family podiatrist.

He X-rayed my foot after noting the swelling around my ankle and diagnosed me with Achilles Tendonitis. When I mentioned that

I had recently run a very hilly 10K, he congratulated me on my race and ordered me to avoid running for at least two weeks.

While I recognized that this injury and its recovery time weren't as serious as when I broke my foot, I was frustrated to be sidelined again. I had a 5K on my calendar for early May and questioned whether I would be able to run it or have to cancel.

I spent the next two weeks swimming, using the elliptical, and training with Jeff. He believed I hadn't actually injured myself in a fall but had simply pushed too hard while training for the 10K.

By allowing myself time to heal properly, I was able to participate in the Montefiore Home Run 5K in May as planned. I ran it with my cousin and friend, Adam, in 31:37, but I felt discouraged trying to match my previous race times, not fully appreciating that I was a year older and had just recovered from an overuse injury.

I finished 7th out of 17 in my age group and 84th out of 217 overall, so I wasn't too upset, though it wasn't a personal best.

After we finished, I stayed with Adam to watch the awards ceremony. His father placed in the top three for his age group, which was inspiring, but even more impressive was a 96-year-old woman being awarded for setting an unverified record in the 100 and 200 meter dashes for women aged 95 to 99.

As she waved to the crowd, I told myself that I wanted to be her when I grew up.

In June, I ran my third Gathering Place Race for the Place, this time in the 50–54 age group. The same course, a different race shirt, but just as meaningful an experience. On a very humid morning, I finished in 29:00:5 and placed 374th out of 2600 overall. There were moments when I had to slow down and walk for a few seconds, but I quickly got back into my running groove and pushed through to honor the many cancer warriors and survivors in my life.

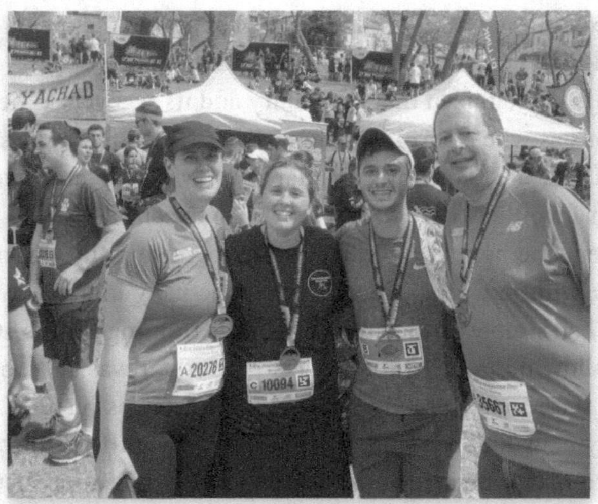

© 2018 Zev Weiss

My next big race was on Father's Day, June 17, and I did this 5-miler with my friends Frankie and Miki. Frankie was just recovering from a hip injury, and we all agreed to take it easy, running when we felt like it and walking when necessary. It was the first race where I focused on enjoying the experience with my friends rather than checking my time and pace.

Despite the heat, the course was beautiful as we ran and walked through Shaker Heights and the Van Aken area. After the first two miles, Frankie felt it was too much, so we switched to walking. Occasionally, we tried to run, but I knew not to push Frankie, who was in pain.

As we finished mile 4, a policeman drove by and asked if we needed help getting back, but we assured him we were fine. We made our way to the finish line, holding hands and cheering with joy as we crossed it. We didn't care that we were the last finishers; we finished the race feeling proud and jubilant.

A few hours later, I checked the results and noticed our names weren't listed. I was upset and promptly emailed the race director, explaining that I had run with a friend who was recovering from an injury. He replied, saying there was a one-hour cutoff, and we had finished in one hour, ten minutes, and twenty-three seconds. He agreed to add our names to the results page, which made me feel I had advocated well for myself and my friends.

On July 9, I swam a full mile! While it may not seem impressive to others, it was a significant achievement for me, as I had been working for months to relearn the swim strokes I once knew well as a child. I didn't yet realize that all this swimming would come in handy seven months later when I participated in the JCC indoor triathlon.

The rest of the summer had me training for my second River Run Half. I'm not sure what possessed me to sign up, especially considering my poor finish at the Rite Aid in 2017. My older son, Seth, was visiting for the race weekend and promised to run with me, so I figured, "Why not?!" I felt a bit guilty about him having to slow down for my pace, but I was excited at the prospect of running together.

Training this time proved much more challenging than for my previous halves. I found myself doing timed runs, speed intervals, and long runs to prepare for race day, but my mojo was lacking. I did many of my long runs indoors, which isn't ideal for an undulating course. When I did run outside, I would run a bit and then switch to walking, which wasn't an effective way to train.

Don't get me wrong—my paces were still strong, but looking back at my Runkeeper notes, I would see many runs marked with an "okay" description. My Instagram posts during that training period included phrases like "I didn't pay attention to the pace," "I pushed through," and "I tried not to think about the time." Those reflected my nearly 50-year-old body, and I truly meant them, as I had transitioned from being a runner obsessed with time and pace to one who runs simply for the joy of it.

I can now see that I was losing my motivation that summer while training for the River Run.

I ran the Bellefaire JCB 5K with Frankie in my old neighborhood of University Heights. We completed it in 33:46 and enjoyed every moment.

It's September 9, and Seth and I get a ride with my friend Dina and her family to the River Run starting line parking lot. We arrived with plenty of time to use the restroom several times, and during one visit, Dina interviewed me for her Instagram vlog!

Showers and storms were predicted for that morning, so I brought a rain poncho, but Seth insisted I take it off before we started the race since it was quite humid. I aimed to run the race with 9–9:30 minute mile splits and had told Seth that no matter how much I complained about aches and pains, he couldn't let me give in to my mental monster telling me 'I can't' or 'this is too hard.'

By mile 8, however, I was feeling a blister on my right foot, and my heel was really achy, so I switched to walking. Seth tried hard to coach and encourage me to run, but I resisted. Unbeknownst to me, Jeff and his wife, Mirvat, were standing on a bridge overlooking the mile 9 marker and saw me saying something to Seth as we passed. In Jeff's words, 'I was yelling at Seth.'

For the rest of the run, I ran whenever I could and walked for about 30 seconds occasionally, but our splits remained steady at a 10–11 minute pace. We finished in 2:15:26—a PR for me! Gary had driven to the West Side to meet us at the finish.

I took a few days off from running and focused on swimming, easy walking, the elliptical, and training with Jeff. Once I resumed running, my paces were steady and strong, and I felt that 50 was the new 30.

About two weeks before my 50th birthday, I was interviewed about my running journey on the *Run Buzz* podcast. The co-hosts asked me how I got into running and what my hopes and dreams were for the future. They inquired if I planned to run a full marathon since I had already completed three half marathons, but I was adamant that a full marathon was not on my goals list. I also stated I would never do a Spartan race, even though Jeff frequently suggested it as a future goal.

While in Israel for the Jewish holidays, I turned 50, and we moved into our new apartment. The gym in our complex wasn't ready yet, so I bought a three-month membership at a nearby mall gym for my runs, elliptical, and TRX workouts. I couldn't train with Jeff during my trips to Israel since I thought there was no way to train virtually. I brought workouts he created for me so I could train on my own and stay active.

Three weeks after my 50th birthday, I ran my first race in the 50–54 age group. It was the Beechbrook 5K, the same course as my very first race. I finished this one in 29:01, managing to shave off a good four minutes, though it felt hillier than the first time. I came to this race alone, ran it solo, and crossed the finish line to a crowd of strangers, but it was a great race nonetheless.

Over the next few months, I attended spin classes at the JCC two to three times a week and increased my running. Jeff introduced me to the track as a new way to improve my running, but I didn't love it. I found it frustrating to weave in and out of lanes while passing other walkers and runners, and I was terrified of crashing into the corners. I doubted that anyone had ever crashed into a corner at the JCC, but you know me.

Jeff had me do intervals around the track, running three laps and walking two. I went from dreading it to tolerating it, and eventually, I actually enjoyed it. I believe that all my track work made me a better runner. I continued to do speed intervals on the treadmill, pushing for challenging yet achievable paces.

I finished off 2018 by signing up for the 2019 Jerusalem Marathon 10K and the Spartan Sprint with Jeff in the fall. My paces going into the new year were steady, and I was feeling strong and (gulp!) lean. Things were looking good!

CHAPTER 5

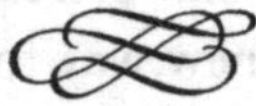

YOU WANT ME TO DO WHAT?!

The early months of 2019 were spent training for my second Jerusalem Marathon 10K, running in the 9-to-10-minute mile range. I relied on the treadmill for my training runs more than I should have, but at least I was getting them done. I resumed long runs and interval training on the track, along with speed and hill workouts.

I aimed to diversify my cardio activities, so in addition to running, I used the elliptical and Stairmaster and attended spinning classes whenever possible. I even joined a few "gentle yoga" classes at the JCC, probably lowering the average age by twenty or thirty years! The gym in our apartment complex in Israel unofficially opened in late January, and I was the first to use the equipment.

In February, I began training with Jeff for my first Spartan race, scheduled for September 8. I had insisted for a long time that I wouldn't participate in such an event, but I eventually threw caution to the wind and signed up. I didn't want to get muddy, crawl under barbed wire, or jump over a fire pit, knowing I would likely end up cut and burned. Yet, something compelled me to give it a try and join Jeff, putting my worries aside.

We signed up for the Spartan Sprint—a 5K trail run with 20 challenging obstacles. If you fail to complete an obstacle, you must do 30 burpees! We had over six months to prepare, which I needed to adequately train for the obstacles.

Jeff incorporated Spartan-like activities into our sessions, such as having me carry 20- or 25-pound saddlebags over my shoulder while walking across the fitness center and up and down the stairs. I felt like I was on *The Biggest Loser*, hoisting the saddlebags and recalling how I had carried that extra weight before committing to fitness and cleaner eating. He also had me use the rope pull machine, which would be useful on race day with the Hercules Hoist obstacle.

As for my second Jerusalem Marathon 10K, it was a different experience than the previous year but still enjoyable and fulfilling. Gary walked the 5K while Yonatan ran his own 10K and Seth ran the half. I had the pleasure of meeting his girlfriend (now wife) the night before and felt ready for the race. The course was the same as the previous year, which I appreciated, and I loved seeing so many friends before and after the race.

The only downside was that my 50-year-old hips didn't appreciate the run. Looking back, I realize I should have trained more outdoors instead of solely on the treadmill, and I wasn't diligent about stretching before and after my runs. This run felt significantly harder, and I found myself walking the last kilometer—until a fellow runner encouraged me in Hebrew to run to the finish. I asked him in Hebrew if Jeff had sent him to motivate me, and he looked confused before running off to finish his race. I jogged to the finish line and saw my time was 1:07:51, which wasn't too bad despite having to walk at the end.

I took a few days to rest before resuming my running. I didn't like the idea of inactivity now that I enjoyed working out. I did take a break, starting with a brisk walk on the treadmill the Sunday after the race and then a 20-minute workout on the elliptical the following day.

While flying back to Cleveland, I realized I actually needed that time to recover. My body was tired after the race, and I needed to give it time to heal. Next up was training for a 10K in May! Timed runs, track intervals, and mile repeats were on my training agenda.

I decided to start a blog on March 22, naming it *"You Want Me*

To Do What?!" The title came to me quickly, as it was a phrase I often thought—or said—while working with Jeff. A Spartan race? A half marathon? A 5K? Many of the challenges in my training pushed me out of my comfort zone and into seemingly impossible territory.

In an Instagram post, I shared, *"It's not just the big things we get to celebrate."* I wrote the blog to document my fitness journey and how I transitioned from a sedentary wife and mother of five to a 50-year-old quasi-athlete.

I embraced the challenges that Jeff presented, often responding with an *"Um, what?!"* In April, I participated in a push-up challenge, starting with 20 push-ups on April 1 and increasing the count daily until I reached 60. A few months prior, I couldn't do more than two "real" push-ups—but by April 1, I was somewhat of a pro.

In June, I was a solo participant in a 30-day burpee challenge, although I mistakenly believed it ended after 28 days! That challenge significantly improved my burpee ability, which would prove useful for the Spartan race.

On April 7, I ran the Towpath Trilogy 3 Mile and placed first in my age group. Yes, you read that right—I placed first! It didn't matter that there were only five others in my age group.

I enjoyed the ride to and from the race, courtesy of the Fixler family, and I can even brag that I finished before Dina and her husband finished their race! (To be fair, they ran a half marathon, but who's keeping track?!)

I completed this race in 26:33, finishing 18th out of 96 overall. Though there were no prizes for top finishers in each age group, I was thrilled with my time and the fact that I PLACED FIRST IN MY AGE GROUP!!!

I didn't need a medal that day. I celebrated the victory of being 50 and having started running just four years prior, accomplishing something I never thought possible.

I began acclimating to the track workouts. Despite my initial fears and resentment, I realized that the track work was helping me build speed. On April 15, I ran my first full mile on the track. Then I did it a second time!

I had run a mile plenty of times on the road, trails, and treadmill, but I had never completed a full mile on the track. I recalled running six consecutive laps, which equaled a half mile, and thought that was a significant accomplishment!

On that April 15 morning, Jeff and I reviewed the workout plan, and I heard him say I would be running a mile on the track—twice. I looked at him in sheer panic and disbelief, as I often do when he suggests something seemingly out of reach. I couldn't believe he expected me to run an entire mile, and that he would be timing me AND I would be doing it a second time?!

Before I could grab my purse and flee the gym, he told me to get started on the circuit. I completed the first circuit twice—15 mid rows with the TRX, 25 modified push-ups, and 25 squats—followed by that dreaded mile.

I ran 12 laps around the track, with people walking and jogging alongside me. Jeff timed me as I completed each lap, and I'll admit I gave him the finger after the first count. After that initial lap, I tuned everything out and focused on finishing each lap. I completed it in 8:36, and then we walked slowly around the track to recover. (Well, I needed to recover.)

During the walk, Jeff gave me a pep talk about how well I did. I repeated the TRX/push-up/squat circuit downstairs and then ran the second mile, although I was a bit slower this time. Despite feeling taxed, I pushed to finish the mile in under 9 minutes. I completed that 12th lap in 8:59, still under 9 minutes!

I was on such a high afterward, reveling in the glory of having accomplished something I never had before, and I did it... twice!

In my training sessions with Jeff, I grew stronger every month. Whether it was pushing 160–220 pounds on the glute press machine or swinging a 20-pound kettlebell, I enjoyed everything that strength training offered—losing body fat, gaining strength, reducing my chances of osteoporosis, and improving my posture.

May 19 was my second Cleveland Rite Aid Marathon 10K, and this time, I ran without Jeff as my running buddy and source of motivation. Gary once again got up at dawn to drive me downtown, see me off at the starting line, and take a picture as I crossed the finish line.

I hadn't slept well the night before, but I didn't feel sleep-deprived that race day morning. When I saw the forecast, I tried not to overanalyze it, especially since I didn't understand what a combination of 68 degrees, 74% humidity, and a 60 dew point meant.

Standing at the starting line, I felt excited to race, and surprisingly, I wasn't nervous about running alone. (Well, I guess I wasn't really alone since there were 15,000 other participants!) A boy on crutches stood next to me as we waited, and while I didn't know his story, he looked just as excited to start the race.

My plan was to aim for splits in the 9-minute mile range to PR from my first 10K, which was 57:03. Getting across the starting line and through the first mile took some time due to the large crowd. The first three miles went well, and the course was mostly flat, but I remembered from running this course two years earlier that a big hill was coming.

I reminded myself not to worry about the hills until I reached them, and then I would deal with them as best as I could. By the time I reached the first hill, it was getting more humid, and I realized I would have to mix fast walking and running to get up it, rather than running and exhausting myself with a few miles left.

At that point, I hoped to finish in an hour since a PR was definitely out of reach. I saw the last of the hills by the bridge where I had collapsed from heat exhaustion during my second half marathon, and in that moment, I just ran for it, determined to get across the bridge and make it to the finish line, which was only a quarter mile away.

I saw on my watch that an hour had already passed, so that second goal was out of reach. I just wanted to finish, having done my best under challenging circumstances. And I did.

My finish time was 1:02:46, placing 214 out of 1,133 in my gender group, 17 out of 94 in my age group, and 549 out of 1,961 overall. I was okay with that.

While running, I thought of my mantra: *I get to do this.* Yes, I can do this, but I am also fortunate to have two feet that allow me to run when others are not as fortunate or choose not to.

Remember the boy in the wheelchair at the starting line? Later that day, I read on a local news website that he was hit by a car while riding his bicycle the previous week and had broken his ankle. He had planned on running the 10K with his fellow high school students, and after his accident, his only concern was participating in the race. He was pushed in a wheelchair for most of the race and finished the last quarter mile on crutches.

I also learned later that a 22-year-old woman had died in the hospital after collapsing at the race.

How could I possibly doubt myself or complain about my time when I was healthy and blessed to run? I finished in the top 25th percentile overall! I outran 77 people in my age group and 919 other women in the 10K. I finished, and I can honestly say I was pleased.

Our family drove to Detroit for Memorial Day Weekend to celebrate my niece's wedding. I hadn't run all week to allow time for recovery, but by that Friday, I was ready to run. I decided to do an easy run around my parents' suburb, which included rolling hills on a mile-long street.

I had never considered running in their area since running outside on hills felt so out of my realm. That morning, I ran up and down a few streets, then tackled the street with the rolling hills, and you know what? It felt totally fine, and I averaged a 9:03 minute mile pace!

I ran my fourth Gathering Place Race for the Place 5K on June 2, this time in honor of Josh Hurand, a dear family friend. Josh's sister is married to Gary's youngest brother, and he had been battling advanced prostate cancer like a true warrior.

This 5K always reminds me of the faces of many friends and family members who have battled cancer — my grandmothers, great-aunts, and friends. Many did not win the battle, while others have survived and are living their lives as best they can.

I ran this 5K, refusing to give in to any discomfort along the way. I imagined Josh smiling ear to ear, as I had always seen him. I sent healing thoughts to him and prayers of strength to his loved ones, making this run about something more than the official time or fancy medal. This run was about perseverance, resilience, and endurance, and all I wanted were those three things for Josh and every person battling cancer. I finished that race in 27:26, placing 245 out of 1,377 overall.

With those races behind me, I focused more on running outside and less on the treadmill. I ran my first-ever trail run with Jeff on June 5, and it was everything he had said it would be and more! I loved running on the towpath and trails and appreciated how that terrain felt compared to the treadmill and roads.

I admit I was a bit apprehensive leading up to that first trail run. I overthought things—how to dress, what if I tripped and fell, how humid it would be at 4 in the afternoon, and how I would get through 3 miles. All that fear and nervousness faded as I drove to the trail park that morning. I felt excited about trying it out.

I knew enough from Jeff that trail running was very different and involved more leg work than running on the treadmill or roads. I also knew this would be an important part of my training for the Spartan race in September, making it the first of many trail runs.

During the run, I either ran alongside Jeff or just behind him, and he only had to warn me once to let him lead and keep enough distance between us. I paid extra attention to the trails, watching for loose branches and muddy areas, and I tried to follow Jeff's directions to keep my body upright and my feet off the ground.

He chose a mostly flat trail with just a few minor elevation bumps, but I kept a steady pace and determination. The run was just under 3 miles in 28 minutes and seven seconds, and I managed negative splits, meaning each mile got faster.

My legs got a good workout, and I felt tired but energized afterward. I was so glad I did it and felt like I had accomplished something big. I was pleasantly surprised when I saw the calorie burn on Runkeeper—411 calories in less than 30 minutes?! I wouldn't get those kinds of results on a treadmill!

My son and his girlfriend got engaged in mid-June that year, giving me extra motivation to keep my weight in check. While in Israel, I tried to run outside as much as possible and manage the stony pavement and hilly roads. Back home in Cleveland, I ran through Shaker Lakes and Beachwood Park, and even ran with a friend in South Chagrin Reservation.

I ran my first trail race at the Full Moon Trail Series 3-miler on July 17. About 180 other runners lined up, and I was determined not to focus on my time since it was my first race and there was nothing to compare it to. All I knew going into this race was that there'd be a big staircase to climb in the first mile—and that it would be really humid, even at 6 PM. Jeff offered to start the race with me and then do his own thing, which I appreciated. I was grateful for his presence, knowing I wasn't alone with so many others around.

They started the race in waves, allowing groups of 10–20 runners at a time to prevent congestion on the trails. We were in the later group, which was fine; I needed some time to mentally prepare and get excited about stepping out of my comfort zone.

The first mile went well, and Jeff ran with me until we reached the staircase. I told him to go ahead, and I'd see him later. Everyone, and I mean everyone, was walking up the stairs and taking their time, so even if I wanted to run, I couldn't get around them. Walking up the stairs slowed my time and pace, but I knew I had to save energy for when I reached the top and could resume running.

The second mile was slower, mostly due to other runners walking on the narrower trails, making it difficult to weave around them. I ran when I could and walked when I couldn't, and before I knew it, I was nearing the third mile. There was a lot of mud and debris on the ground, and I did my best to stay steady and avoid slipping, especially when I had to jog down a long staircase.

This trail race experience was something I had never envisioned doing, but I learned through my fitness journey that there are countless possibilities. You just have to find the desire within yourself to try, do your best, and believe in yourself.

I finished the race in 34:02 and knew I would be doing many more trail runs.

Swimming became an option for cross-training when I didn't feel like using the elliptical or couldn't make it to my Friday morning spin class. I had been swimming regularly after a long hiatus, but as I started doing more 10Ks and half marathons, running took precedence.

I found myself really enjoying the weekly swim workouts that gradually increased my lap count, and the previous summer, I managed to swim a full mile! That was huge for me! Keep in mind that I hadn't swum a lap since my preteens or worn a bathing suit in public! I never did it for time or speed; it was all about having the right form and enjoying a form of exercise that was out of my comfort zone.

Wearing a bathing suit in public had always been an issue for me. I was ashamed of how I looked and had avoided sitting by a pool during my adult life. When I took up swimming, I felt discomfort walking out of the women's locker room into the pool area for the first time, but I realized everyone else was swimming and not paying attention to me. If they were, they needed to focus on their own forms and not drown. Swimming laps made me feel both energized and spent.

In mid-July, I celebrated my fifth active anniversary, as I called it. Five years after deciding to be more physically active and conscious of my eating, I was doing things I couldn't imagine doing five years earlier. I could barely manage a lunge when I first started working out with Jeff, and five years later, I was lunging with a TRX while holding a knee lift in between.

I learned how to do a proper burpee, which will come in handy for my Spartan in September. Who would have imagined I'd be training for that, knowing how much I dislike getting dirty and how far out of my comfort zone it is?

When I committed to a healthier me five years ago, I didn't know what I expected to gain. I was a wife and mother of five, so engrossed in their lives that I didn't take time for myself or make myself a priority. I was out of shape, both physically and mentally, and I knew I had to change.

As happy as I was with my decision to be more physically fit and active, I felt increasingly defeated by the numbers on the scale. I was obsessed with it, plain and simple. In the past year, I had seen my body change for the better, thanks to my improved diet and workout routine. My legs were getting more muscular, which I noticed in my reflection at the JCC every morning. I got excited as I saw my knees losing the flab that had surrounded them for so long and a shape beginning to form.

Yet I couldn't see past the number on the scale, and as it increased over time, I doubted myself and everything I was doing regarding my eating and workouts. I resembled a deer caught in headlights on the first training session of each month when Jeff weighed me and took my measurements. I hesitated to weigh in at Weight Watchers during that time, continuing a game I played for three years. If I saw a number I didn't like, I would skip my Weight Watchers meeting until I saw a "better" number, but I never thought to do that with my assessments with Jeff.

I would nervously get on the scale for him, worried about the number, but then I would see the measurements tell a story of my progress. How did I let things get to this point? I was in better shape at 50 than ever. I tried to take a break from weighing myself at home, but that didn't last long, and the rollercoaster ride with the scale continued. I had too many mind games: "I can't eat Chinese food for dinner since I'm getting weighed tomorrow, and the sodium will kill me," or "I have to amp up my workout since I'm getting measured tomorrow."

Deep down, I knew I had to stop letting that number dictate my success. I could see my progress when my doctor told me at my yearly physical that he was proud of my hard work, when I finished the 5K, and when others said I inspired them. I wanted to be remembered for taking charge of my health, not for the weight I was supposed to be according to my BMI. No one was judging me for my weight, so I needed to stop doing it to myself.

As the date of the Spartan approached, I was doing more and more training to prepare. I'm sure I looked like a circus act when Jeff had me stand on a plyo box, step onto a resistance band, and move up and down to mimic a pull-up. I walked around the JCC fitness center carrying a 35-pound weighted ball. I was getting there, but Jeff felt I needed to practice wall climbing and conquer my fear of heights, so we met on a Sunday afternoon at Play: CLE, an indoor adventure sports center in Avon.

I didn't know what to expect from this facility, but I certainly didn't expect to see an ambulance pull up and EMTs attend to a young girl who had injured herself in a fall! I knew I had to face my fear of heights to tackle the Spartan race obstacles, and this was the place to do it. Before I knew it, I was harnessed up and climbing a two-story ladder with Jeff right behind me. (The harness would prevent me from falling if I slipped off an obstacle, but I didn't feel any better wearing it.) I had to walk across a ladder from one station to another without anything to hold onto. I had to step onto posts that were quite a distance apart and ensure both feet were in place.

Oh, and there was a zip line. My older son had done it many times without hesitation, but I was not so courageous! I knew there wouldn't be any zip lining at the Spartan race, but my Spartan coach insisted I give it a try. I tried many times, standing at the top of the line, thinking I was ready to step off and start the ride, but then I panicked. After six or seven attempts, I finally took the leap, closed my eyes, and flew across to the landing. I can't remember if I thanked the female staffer who untangled me, but I believe I hugged her!

I genuinely attempted the climbing wall and made it halfway up, but when I saw how high it was, I gave up. The two hours we spent there helped me conquer some fears, and I have no regrets.

On August 4, I participated in the Hofbrau 5K in downtown Cleveland with my oldest child, Yaffa. It was a dream come true to do this race together, just the two of us—and a few thousand other people. We had initially planned to run/walk it, as she had been following a training plan for a few weeks before the race. However, our plans changed on race morning when she woke up feeling nauseous. We ended up walking the entire race, which I was fine with, along with our finishing time of 51:19. A few weeks later, she discovered that she was pregnant with her now five-year-old twins!

In August, my running paces slowed to the 10–11 minute mile range. I participated in the Full Moon Trail Series 4-mile race at Bedford Reservation, finishing in 44:18. As I did more races, I grew accustomed to driving myself to and from them, not wanting to make Gary feel obligated to take me. He continued to be a great source of support and encouragement, but I couldn't ask him to stand around for hours every time I raced on a hot summer evening or early Sunday morning.

I blinked, and it was September 8, also known as the Spartan

Sprint in Brooklyn, Michigan. Having grown up in the Great Lakes State, I was shocked to learn that Brooklyn was over two hours away from my hometown. The day had finally arrived, and I was living it in what felt like an out-of-body experience.

Once I signed up for the race, I felt compelled to share my intentions on Facebook and Instagram to make it feel more real. By putting it out there, I held myself accountable and couldn't back out, no matter how many times I considered it. The people in my life looked at me with wonder and surprise—not doubt about my ability, but with the same expression they had when I first took up running.

I often questioned why I was doing this, sometimes in exasperation and sometimes in jest—why was I putting myself out there, knowing I wouldn't be able to do everything? I worried about getting hurt and dirty, and I was concerned about climbing high ladders. I was excited to try something I never imagined doing, but I was still scared and nervous.

During the three-hour drive from Cleveland to Brooklyn, with Jeff driving and his wife, Mirvat, as our photographer and cheerleader, I resolved to embrace the mud in the dunk wall and the heights of the ladders, knowing it would be fun. It felt a bit strange to have Jeff hoist me over the four-, five-, and six-foot walls, but we were a team. We tackled some obstacles together while dividing others based on my comfort level, letting him handle the ones I knew I couldn't attempt.

I was fine with the heavy carries and was told by my Spartan partner that I aced the Hercules Hoist. I offered encouragement as Jeff tackled the monkey bars and rope climbs that I wisely avoided. I took my time rolling around on the grass, just inches from the barbed wire, and emerged snag-free.

The most challenging obstacle was the Slip Wall, which I had to ascend and descend right after the dunk wall. Picture this: I willingly walked into muddy water, closed my eyes, and dunked myself under a wall without hitting it. Once I surfaced, I had to find my way to dry land while trying to regain my composure.

I then faced the Slip Wall, with Jeff halfway up, urging me to follow him. I realized that as long as he was doing the obstacle, I didn't necessarily have to, but Jeff insisted. I remember stepping onto the wall with my muddy shoes, grabbing a rope connected to the top, and starting to climb. I slipped a few times but pushed myself to keep going. Jeff encouraged me from the top, promising to help me up.

With him gripping my left shoulder and a fellow Spartan grabbing my right, I felt uncertain but determined to reach the top. I'm not sure if it was their encouragement or something within me that propelled me over the wall, but I made it. Jeff often reminds me that when I realized I had reached the top, it was a defining moment.

I had conquered something significant, similar to when I jumped over a pit of fire just before crossing the finish line. Jeff and I finished in 1:17:32, and we didn't do a single burpee!

I can't count how many times I questioned why I chose to do this race. It wasn't on my bucket list, and it was far outside my comfort zone. But during the race and in the hours afterward, I found my answer. I may have signed up for it, but the race chose me.

I had spent so much of my life doubting myself and my abilities, saying I couldn't. I never saw myself as a runner. For decades, I watched others run outside, wishing I could join them, but fearing how foolish I would look or how I might injure myself.

In July 2014, I decided to start my fitness and wellness journey. I began by turning a walk on a treadmill into a jog, then a run, and before I knew it, I had signed up for a 5K.

Entering the Spartan race, I was filled with doubts and fears, but crossing the starting line, I felt determined to enjoy it, make the most of it, and tackle the obstacles I could manage. I wouldn't feel like a failure for skipping an obstacle that posed an injury risk, nor would I attempt one that was beyond my capabilities.

When I pushed myself upward and let Jeff and our fellow racer help me over the climb wall, I experienced an ah-ha moment. Despite the physical struggle and my initial urge to give up, I knew I had the encouragement and support to help me reach the top. Once I realized I could do it, I gave it my all.

I reached the top, got myself down, and resumed my run, filled with a sense of pride and accomplishment that had never come easily to me. That was when I understood why I needed to do this.

The old feeling of "I can't" was replaced by "heck yeah… I can." That was the answer to my constant questioning, the reason I sought, and my defining moment.

Once I got over the shock of completing the Spartan race, I mentioned to Jeff that I was considering doing an indoor triathlon down the road. Every February, our JCC hosts this event, but I had never really paid much attention to the posters and ads promoting it in past years. It was something I could never see myself doing, yet it wasn't an impossible goal. I could run, spin, and swim — just not all simultaneously and in a timed format.

The indoor triathlon would have me swimming as many laps as I could in 15 minutes, spinning as many miles as possible in 20 minutes, and running as many laps around the track in 20 minutes. It all seemed overwhelming, and of course, I had many questions. How would I manage to change out of my bathing suit and dry off in time for the spin portion? How could I spin without changing the resistance on the bike? How would I run for 20 minutes straight on the track?

I asked a few people who had done the race in previous years, and they all assured me I would be fine. As I thought more about the triathlon, I figured, "Why not?!" It was a goal outside my comfort zone, but one I could work toward and achieve. I signed up for the event, deciding to do it because it was different, without setting a specific time or pace goal for myself.

Jeff thought it was a great idea and helped me create a training plan that included weekly spin classes, lots of running on the track, and plenty of swimming. I still didn't love running on the track, but I knew those workouts were necessary for my triathlon preparation. There were days when Jeff included track workouts in my training sessions, and days when I had to do it on my own.

Many mornings, I didn't feel like it, but I knew I had to push through. I became adept at using my stopwatch to track my laps, despite occasionally hitting the reset or stop button by mistake. Sometimes, I faced an inner battle, with one side urging me to push through the run and the other reminding me to simply do my best.

Quitting was never an option, though there were moments when I had to silence that inner voice telling me I'd had enough.

Two weeks after the Spartan, I participated in the University Heights 5K Inaugural Beautiful Run. It was held just outside the school building where my kids had attended preschool and grade school, so I hadn't seen the newly renovated building and beautiful park that surrounded it.

While waiting for the race to start, a fellow runner approached me, saying he recognized me from my posts on the Diz Runs Facebook page! The city mayor greeted all the runners and announced the start, and off we went, running through the streets of University Heights. Though I lived only two miles from the race course, I had never had the opportunity to explore those streets and see how beautiful the neighborhood was. I completed the 5K in 28:56.

Another month, another fitness challenge. October's challenge called for 25 push-ups and 50 squats each day, with the real challenge being to increase the count daily to ultimately reach 50 push-ups and 100 squats by the month's end.

A very wise person once told me that you never do a Spartan race just once; you do it, then set a bigger goal and keep going. I thought I was content with my one Spartan. I had trained as best I could for that race, didn't have to do any burpees, and even completed some obstacles I hadn't expected to conquer. I was sure this was a one-and-done experience and was happy to return to focusing on my strength and cardio.

Apparently, my coach/teammate thought differently. Recalling the rush of adrenaline and feeling of triumph when I crossed the finish line—something I had never experienced in any other race—I agreed to do another Spartan.

On November 18, I signed up for the 2020 Spartan in Ohio as part of Team Why Nots?! The name perfectly captured my fitness journey. Many people had asked me over the years why I took up running and why I subjected myself to the risk of hurting my knees and hips. Why did I take my fitness so seriously? My answer to all those questions was, "Why not?!"

For most of my life, I had doubted myself and didn't believe in my potential. During my training for that first Spartan, I often asked Jeff why I was doing it. Each time, I was told I would figure it out, and that clarity came when I reached the top of the climbing wall. I could have given up each time I slipped, but I didn't, and with the help of some Spartan friends, I made it to the top and continued my race.

I was ready to do it again on May 31! When I told Gary I would be doing another Spartan, he looked both confused and proud. What had happened to the girl he married thirty years ago?!

CHAPTER 6

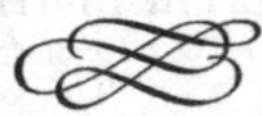

RUNNING TOWARD SOMETHING

I rang in 2020 riding high from seeing my son marry his bride just a few days earlier, on December 30. I kept up with my exercise routine in the week after his wedding but also allowed myself some days to relax without working out—which was unusual for me. Those rest days helped me recharge, and, surprisingly, I didn't feel guilty for giving myself grace.

I started the new year by making a list of races that appealed to me, along with a list of a few races I had already signed up for. I even included a fall half marathon in my wish list, despite having previously declared I would never run another half. I went so far as to look up a few half marathon training plans and printed them out in case Jeff needed a break from creating his own.

Making a wish list greatly improved my mindset, which had been lacking. Somewhere along the way, I had convinced myself that I couldn't surpass a three-mile barrier in my running. I would run three miles and then stop, believing I couldn't do any more.

By creating a wish list, I knew I needed to change my mindset and work toward more than a three-mile run. I was fully capable of running three and a half miles, four miles, or more—I just needed a mental shift to think positively.

I crafted my own training plan that included interval runs and easy runs ranging from three and a half to five miles. I ensured I included a rest day, along with my two training days with Jeff and two cross-training days.

I officially became a triathlete on February 9. It sounds impressive, so I won't downplay what I accomplished to reach this point or what I achieved at the event itself. I had joined the JCC board in the summer of 2019 and signed up for the event, feeling like I was contributing.

I swam 17 lengths in 15 minutes and imagined I was in one of Kate's spinning classes during the biking portion. As for the run, I didn't feel as energetic starting out since my legs were tired from all that biking. I began a bit faster for the first three laps, then slowed down, staying in the inside lane and sometimes just following the person ahead of me.

Running for 20 minutes after an intense swim and bike workout was something I'd never done, and again, I won't downplay what I accomplished. I finished the event and was so glad I did, even though my glutes, quads, and every other muscle in my body were screaming.

I stepped out of my comfort zone again when I met up with a fellow runner from a running group I found on Facebook. I don't remember exactly how I discovered the Cleveland MRTT/SRTT group, but once I did, I became an active member, sharing posts about my runs.

This particular runner had posted looking for someone to run with on the East Side of Cleveland, so I privately messaged her, offering to meet up. Alexandra was just getting back into running after having a baby and wanted to run 2–3 miles. I told her I was fine with whatever she wanted to do, planning to get in any extra miles I needed at the gym to complete my six-mile long run that day.

We met on March 1 at Acacia Reservation, the same place where I had broken my foot while running with Jeff. Returning to Acacia that morning brought mixed feelings; I had to be careful not to slip on the ice or snow, but I was confident I could finish this run injury-free.

Alexandra was friendly and sweet, and I really enjoyed running and chatting with her about our running journeys. I managed to stay upright as we navigated patches of snow and ice, and I didn't mind that it was 27 degrees outside.

On March 8, I ran the *Kiss Me I'm A Runner* 5K at Legacy Village with my friend Kimi. She had only recently taken up running in the last few months, and this was her very first race. I didn't care about the time; I was just happy to share the experience with her. This was going to be *her* race.

She had a time in mind, having run on her treadmill many times, but I told her that running outside might increase her pace. We started at the back of the pack, running/walking while enjoying the chance to chat and appreciate the course. I played the role of running coach, occasionally telling her our pace, how far we had gone, and how much was left. Our finish time was 34:43, and she placed 74th out of 160 women!

Then came Covid.

It hit my home state in early March and wasn't going away anytime soon. Schools closed, retail stores shut down, and even the JCC closed. I received an email stating the JCC would be closed through April 5, and I panicked. How would I work out without my favorite treadmill? How could I train with Jeff?

I quickly composed myself; I knew this was temporary and merely an inconvenience. I dusted off the treadmill in my basement and started using it for mile repeats and interval runs, and I bought some weights and a TRX for home training.

Many races transitioned to virtual formats, and several were canceled altogether. There was still hope for two big races scheduled for May, and the Spartan race in Ohio was still happening.

I did a 35-minute timed run with my younger son, Yonatan, at Acacia. We ran at a pace much slower than he was used to, but he was great about sticking to what I could do. It was nice to have some alone time with him and get outside after so many indoor runs.

I continued to follow my training plan for the River Run half marathon, needing the structure even without a race deadline. I returned to running speed and hill intervals, mile repeats, and shakeout runs, where I'd run simply to loosen my legs. My running pace started slipping into the 10-plus minute mile range, and I found myself making excuses when posting on Instagram, like "I wasn't feeling great" or "my hip started to hurt a mile in..."

I met Jeff for a trail run in Rocky River one morning in early April. Just a few steps in, I felt alive and grateful to be back on the trails.

I continued with my strength training, using the TRX I bought for my home gym and following workouts that Jeff wrote out for me or offered through the JCC website. With the JCC closed indefinitely, various personal trainers provided virtual workouts, and I took advantage as much as possible. Whether it was a yoga class or a stability ball workout, I was determined to stay active.

My running pace seemed to return to the nine to ten minute mile range after my twin grandson and granddaughter were born on April 13. My daughter, her husband, and the babies moved into our home for a few weeks, making it somewhat challenging to carve out time for my workouts.

Since starting my fitness journey, I had considered running and working out my "me time." No matter what was happening in my life, I needed that time each day to turn everything off and run, walk, or train to maintain my physical and mental health.

By the beginning of May, races throughout Ohio were either canceled, postponed, or changed to virtual. I began to feel a funk after realizing that the races I had planned to participate in this year were unlikely to happen. The Ohio Spartan race was postponed to mid-July, and it didn't look promising since this race involved a lot of physical contact between runners.

I continued with my running, adhering to my plan to stay accountable. During one of our many runs together, Jeff took a picture of me running on the trails. When I first saw the photo in a text, I cringed, thinking about how terrible I must look, how big my bottom was, and how no matter how much I ran, it remained the same. But then I realized I was running toward something, and Jeff was capturing that moment. It was a fleeting snapshot of my journey.

Here I was, a 51-year-old wife, mother, and grandmother—more athletic and stronger than I had been 20 or 30 years ago! This photo told the story of how I was stepping out of my comfort zone, getting outside, being active, and able to run during a challenging time (Covid). It showed me running toward something—whether it was the parking lot where my car was parked or crossing a stream along the trails—I was running, giving no thought to how I might look.

On May 21, I received an email from Spartan announcing that the Ohio race rescheduled for July 18–19 was officially canceled. I admit I was disappointed but not surprised. I had just stocked up on gloves for the hand-gripping obstacles I planned to tackle, but I knew it would be challenging to race with so much personal contact between competitors.

With the race canceled and my entry deferred until next summer, I decided to stick to my training plan to have something to work toward, even without actual races. I needed the structure of a workout, which would benefit me mentally and physically.

I made a few tweaks when I shared my training plan with Jeff, but overall, it was solid. I implemented what I had learned from him over the years about the various runs that would serve me best. Jeff texted me, expressing how proud he was of my ability and confidence to create my own plan and be the driver of my training rather than the passenger.

With no idea when I would return to the JCC, I started investing in my own gym in the basement. I had a stability ball that needed air, and I added various dumbbells, kettlebells, and slam balls to my collection. I also bought a Bosu trainer and mounted a TRX on the basement ceiling, ensuring I had everything I needed for my workouts with Jeff.

When we began training virtually in late May, I thought it would be easier than working out together in person. No such luck! I bought a tripod for my iPad and positioned it so Jeff could see me as I moved around my basement. He started each session with a quick summary of the planned circuit, to which I would often respond, "Um, excuse me?!" We would then begin, with him watching from his house while I worked out in my basement, ensuring I maintained the correct form. It felt like being in the gym together, even though we were a good 30 minutes apart. These virtual workouts proved just as invigorating and challenging as our in-person sessions.

When I wasn't doing mile repeats or speed intervals on the treadmill, I spent as much time outside as possible, particularly on the trails with Jeff. I became increasingly familiar with the Rocky River Reservation and its various trails, but when he introduced me to the Brecksville Reservation in late May, I was hooked on trail running.

While descending a hill and stepping onto a new trail, I missed a step and fell. I felt my bottom hit the ground and skinned my knee in the process. Covered in dirt and debris, I got back up, dusted myself off, and continued running. I felt some stinging from my knee and noticed blood trickling down my leg, but I felt like a total badass. I had stopped my fall and avoided further injury by using my hands—skinned knee and bruised bottom aside. I got back on my feet and kept running.

On my drive home, I reflected on how just a year ago, Jeff had introduced me to trail running, insisting I would love it. After our first run in Rocky River, I was sold and wondered why I hadn't tried it sooner. Don't get me wrong—I didn't love running through mud and dirtying my shoes, but with each trail run, I learned to embrace it.

I had to focus on staying upright while running downhill to avoid slipping and mastering walking up hills with strides instead of trying to run and wipe out. I loved seeing the waterfalls and crossing bridges over streams. Each trail run that summer and beyond made me feel one with nature, allowing me to forget about tracking my time and pace. My focus was solely on every step I took to finish intact.

During my annual checkup in June, my (now former) doctor asked what I did for exercise. I told her I ran three to four times a week and trained with Jeff twice a week. I thought I had made it clear that I ran 12 to 15 miles a week, but she again asked if I was okay with my activity level.

I didn't think much about it when I repeated my answer, but a few hours later, I began to wonder why she was questioning me. I started to feel defensive and questioned whether my activity was enough. I decided to step up the intensity of my runs and workouts, even though I had nothing specific to train for.

(Side note: I switched doctors soon after that appointment, and my current internist frequently tells me how impressed he is with my running and workouts.)

In mid-June, Jeff and I did a six-plus-mile run in Brecksville, starting at the nature center and heading down to the towpath that led to the Carriage Trail. The first mile or so was just basic pavement alongside the metropark's main road. Once we crossed the bridge by the old train station, we hit the towpath.

We had already run nearly three miles, passing a snapping turtle, a dead squirrel, bikers, and joggers. Jeff had promised me earlier that we would tackle some killer hills, and he delivered! I was ready for the challenge when we reached the Carriage Trail, and he told me to lead the way. I felt like the little engine that could, chugging up the hill before turning around and running back down.

Once back on the towpath, we returned to our starting point at the nature center. Just before reaching the parking lot, we encountered a series of three hills, and I was determined to jog them and finish strong. I jogged up the first hill and resumed running at the top, then walked the second and third hills with strides since I was pretty taxed.

I loved the mix of terrain on this run—the towpath, paved roads, and trails—and I couldn't wait for the next opportunity. That came a week later when I met Jeff for a 10K trail run at Brecksville.

We met at the old train station parking lot and began our run on the towpath for a mile and a half. I recognized certain landmarks from our previous runs before hitting the Carriage Trail. That hill was steep, and this time, we jogged up and continued our run on the trails.

The trails were beautiful, with narrow paths, mud, and roots, yet so peaceful. We ran a few miles before descending the hill and continuing on the towpath back to the train station parking lot. That 10K was unlike any I had done before; it required intense focus and self-encouragement, even when I felt like giving up.

My legs were sore, but in a good way, and I felt as if I had run a marathon.

On a trail run with Jeff in early July, he had me lead instead of staying a few feet behind, as was our usual arrangement. He wanted me to set the pace while keeping my breathing under control. I had never been great at following directions, but the colored signs on the trails helped me navigate. We followed the red trail, and when I was unsure how to proceed, Jeff guided me from a few feet behind.

There were several hills along the way, and I tried to tackle them with shorter strides and synchronized arm movement. I walked up some hills, feeling guilty for not running, but I knew I had to gauge what I could handle. Our second mile was our slowest due to elevation changes, and Jeff paused in the middle to take pictures and snap a photo of me running ahead. For the downhill sections, I moved laterally as Jeff had taught me to avoid slipping.

During training sessions, I never knew what Jeff had planned. Even after six years of working together, he would surprise me, often prompting a response of "You want me to do what?!"—like doing X number of burpees or holding a 2-minute plank. Regardless of his challenges, I knew it would all be beneficial, and I would follow through with whatever he had in store.

One day, he had me do four sets of five squats with the TRX, five high/mid/low rows with the TRX, 12 bicep curls with 10-pound dumbbells, and then inchworm out into a plank and back up. When I first started working out with Jeff, I couldn't do a push-up; I relied on modified push-ups with my feet on the ground. I didn't believe I could perform a "real" push-up. It took time and practice, but I graduated from modified to "real" push-ups!

I stepped out of my comfort zone again on July 5 when I met some runners from the Cleveland MRTT/SRTT group in Aurora. I had become acquainted with a few of the ladies through their posts, but I had never met them in person. (The group met every Sunday morning outside a Walgreens at 7, and I thought it would be fun to run with them.)

Gary was nervous about me going out early to meet total strangers, but I showed him the group chat with our meetup plans. I left my house at 6:15 AM and drove 30 minutes to Aurora. There were eight of us altogether, and everyone was friendly and welcoming as we introduced ourselves.

I started out running with the group leader and two other runners at the front. The pace felt comfortable until the last mile, when I felt I needed to slow down, but I decided to finish the run with this trio. We chatted about our families, where we lived, and how we found the group on Facebook. Being older than most of these women and somewhat of a newbie runner, I wasn't sure if that morning run would be a one-time thing. But any discomfort I felt faded away as I ran with the group and found a common bond in our love of running.

My running paces had slowed down in June and July, but then I bounced back. I was running outside more frequently, which helped me build the endurance I needed to run longer and faster.

Jeff described our run one evening in July as brutal. He warned me it would be the hardest run I'd ever done. If that didn't convince me to join him and his friend, Lisa, on the CVNP Trailhead course at 5 PM, it was over 90 degrees. I brought water for during and after the run, along with some Himalayan salt for much-needed electrolytes.

I kept my eyes on the ground as we began, watching for debris while also looking ahead. A mile and a half in, we reached "dry" land. After a few more miles on the roads, running in the direct humidity, we stopped occasionally to check the maps and ensure we were heading in the right direction.

We got back on the towpath, then hit a field. By then, I was walking more than running. As brutal as this run was, I was determined to see it through, regardless of how long it took or how fast we were going. It was hot and humid, and I no longer had the energy I had at the beginning of our run.

It was a challenge I never would have imagined for myself when I began this fitness journey.

On an early Wednesday morning run in Brecksville, Jeff had me lead the way again. We started on the pavement, encountering three descending hills between the nature center and the bridge parking lot. I maintained a comfortable pace, and whenever I sped up, Jeff reminded me to stay steady for the upcoming hills.

I approached the first hill, trying not to panic, and followed Jeff's advice to take shorter steps to avoid tiring out. Once we crested the hill, I steadied my breathing and prepared for the next. I did the same with the second hill, then braced myself for the third and hardest.

I saw it from a distance and felt a wave of dread, but I knew I could do it. Gradually, I ran up the hill, spotting our finish ahead, and sprinted to the car as Jeff said, "Good job."

I felt more accomplished with this run than I had in a long time. It wasn't about the distance or time; it was about overcoming obstacles—literally and figuratively.

I had never tackled all three hills before, but I did it! I pushed aside fear and discomfort, telling myself I would succeed. Was it hard? Yes. Was it impossible? No. Could I do it again? Absolutely!

I had the best intentions when I decided to work on my hill running the following Monday morning. I wanted to challenge myself and avoid walking up the hills on our trail runs, but I needed practice. I told Jeff I would do the same run in Brecksville as the previous week, omitting that I had done two back-to-back runs two days prior.

I didn't go as far as the train station parking lot since it was getting too hot, and I was tired from running 6.2 miles the day before. All I wanted was to log some miles and run those three hills on the way back to my car.

I saw the first hill and committed to it. I took shorter steps as I ran up and caught my breath at the top. Before reaching the second hill, I decided to call it a day, stopping my watch and switching to a walk. Once home, I did a hill interval run on the treadmill with inclines ranging from 3 to 7%.

I took a nice walk outside on Tuesday before my training session and felt fine. However, those well-meaning intentions came back to haunt me on Wednesday during a pre-run stretch in the train station parking lot.

I felt a tugging in the back of my right knee as Jeff and I left the parking lot and hit the towpath, but I thought little of it. The tugging seemed to fade as we ran our first mile in under ten minutes. I focused on maintaining our pace, knowing we were approaching the Carriage Trail.

The turn came, and there was that hill… I trotted up, thinking we were done at the top, but we still had another hill to conquer. I walked for a few seconds before resuming a trot up the rest. We continued along the trails, turned around, and I thought, "It's all downhill until we get back to the towpath, then about a mile before we're done." Easy, right?

Not quite.

Suddenly, I felt a pop in the back of my right knee where I had felt the tugging, and it screamed at me. I told Jeff something had happened, so we paused while I dealt with the pain radiating down the middle of my calf.

With the run pretty much done, we walked slowly down the hill to the towpath and back to where we started. We talked the whole way back, and I shared with Jeff my efforts to increase my weekly mileage and improve my hill running.

I never thought Monday's run in Brecksville would hinder me. It was just an overuse injury, but I learned my lesson the hard way.

Jeff advised me to ice the area, foam roll, hydrate, and take it easy for the next few days. He made me promise to stick to flatter surfaces for solo runs and leave hill work for our Wednesday trail runs.

It took over a week to recover from that calf strain. I used the foam roller I had bought, did calf raises, iced it, and gave it time to heal. Being sidelined was hardly fun, but I knew I had to wait it out and would be back running soon.

One good thing happened during my recovery — the head of the Cleveland MRTT/SRTT running group asked if I would participate in their member spotlight. I was flattered and shocked by the request and agreed to answer her questions.

If someone had told me five years earlier that I would share my running journey on a Facebook page for mother runners, I would have laughed. I've never been comfortable putting myself out there, especially to strangers, and I've always shied away from being photographed.

I realized that being part of a group meant everyone had a story to share, and perhaps my story could inspire others as theirs had inspired me.

The summer months of 2020 taught me that not having a regular routine meant I could go with the flow. I could run 15–20 miles a week or more, but I had to be mindful not to overdo it and risk another injury. I had to accept some weeks with three runs and others with four, but I would be okay with whatever I could manage. My fitness journey was never meant to be a race.

My running paces dropped to the ten to eleven-minute mile range from August through October, but I was too busy celebrating accomplishments. After returning from a trip in August, I received an email from Runkeeper congratulating me on my 3000th activity! It's hard to believe it all began with a 3.62-mile run with Jeff, just five days before my first 5K race.

It feels like yesterday that Jeff suggested I download the Runkeeper app to track my activities, both indoors and outside. I've grown so much since May 2015. I've had several recovery periods after injuring myself during runs and had to rely on other activities. Over the past few years, I've learned how to handle a day or two of rest when my body signals it needs a break.

I had my redemption run on the Carriage Trail in late August. I had wanted to do it two weeks after straining my calf in July, but then I had a bout of Achilles tendinitis. I needed to ensure I was 100% injury-free before attempting this run again.

He knew I was ready, and I felt prepared. I was determined to follow the course he set for us and complete it all the way back to where we started. The first part of the hills went fine, but I had to switch to a quick walk when we approached the third section. I kept going, and we continued to run to the very top of the trail, where we ran a bit more before starting our descent.

Going down the hills was easier, but I still had to stay in control and make lateral moves to keep my feet planted on the ground. We reached the towpath at the bottom and made our way back to the bridge and then to the parking lot where we began.

As accomplished as I felt after this three-and-a-half-mile run, I experienced a sense of invigoration at the top of the hill when Jeff pointed out where I had strained my calf back in July. Running up those hills was a feat in itself, but revisiting the scene of the injury and finishing the run felt like crossing the finish line of a big race. I didn't get a medal for this run, and I didn't have Gary waiting for me at the end, but I felt redeemed.

In early September, Gary and I returned to Israel for the Jewish holidays and to spend time with three of our kids living there. One afternoon, I listened to a virtual Weight Watchers meeting on how we define ourselves. I participated by listing: *wife, mother, grandmother, daughter, sister, friend, writer, video producer, volunteer... runner.*

After five years of countless runs and races, I still struggled to say the word *runner* out loud. I wasn't an elite runner. I couldn't explain what a Fartlek really meant or what VO2 max was about. I regularly listened to running podcasts, belonged to a few running groups on Facebook, and followed several elite runners on Instagram. Yet, even after more than five years since my first run, I would still blush when someone mentioned my running. I run, yes, but does that make me a runner? I was a runner like Meb and Des, but my paces were different, and I did it for my own reasons.

As we spent more time in Israel, I realized I could work out virtually with Jeff in the gym, just as I had been doing in Cleveland. Our gym allowed residents to reserve an hour slot per Covid protocols, so I claimed the 4–5 PM slot every Tuesday and Thursday! I figured out the best spot for my iPad on the weight rack so that Jeff could see the workout room and ensure my form was correct.

After the first training session, I wondered why we hadn't done this sooner, as it felt like he was right there with me instead of six thousand miles away.

However, while I was excited about our workouts, I didn't have the same drive when it came to my running. I wasn't pushing for more distance or speed, even though I knew I was capable of it. I just lacked the intensity to work harder. I recognized this was a mental hurdle I had faced before, but this time felt different.

In the past, I always had a race or goal to strive for. Thanks to

Covid, I had nothing to train for, and I wasn't sure how to reframe my mindset to regain my motivation for running. I still loved it and wanted to keep going, but something felt off.

I brainstormed a few ideas to rekindle my motivation: create a training plan even without a race, listen to music instead of podcasts on my runs for more stimulation, and use positive self-talk when I felt the urge to stop during a run.

Something eventually clicked, but I can't recall exactly what it was.

I started doing hill interval runs once a week and speed intervals on another day to keep things interesting. Jeff suggested I do a speed run where I sprint fast for 45 seconds, then recover with a walk for three minutes, repeating it six times. I asked if I could jog instead of walk to improve my overall pace, but he insisted on walking for recovery.

I had fast-paced music in my AirPods and got started. I managed those 45-second bursts of speed at a 7:30 to 8-minute mile pace, and when I finished, I felt alive!

Over the next few weeks, I added more intervals and increased the pace of my speed bursts, regaining my momentum.

Once I returned home in mid-October, I compiled a list of goals for the coming months and year. I decided I wanted to train for and beat my personal best of 57:09 in a 10K race—even if no races were planned. I also aimed to do a 5K or two and beat my personal best of 26:48. I knew both goals were ambitious, but I was eager to put in the work to make them a reality.

A third goal was to train for the Spartan race scheduled for June 2021. I knew my running was covered with all the training I did, but I needed to practice the obstacles. Jeff and I discussed going to an indoor obstacle park to improve my wall climbing and grip strength once it reopened. In the meantime, I'd build strength with heavier lifting and work on dynamic movements to prepare for the Spartan.

Our training sessions intensified with plenty of burpees, kettlebell swings, and medicine ball slams. I found myself tiring from the movements but able to keep going from one exercise to the next. It felt more like "oh gosh!" rather than "I can't."

I started logging my runs in a running journal in mid-October. I don't remember who suggested it, but I would like to thank them. I found a running journal online that sold various running accessories and began logging my runs immediately. I felt that tracking my runs would help me find inner motivation by noting the distance, route, pace, and a few comments about how each run went.

The front of the journal featured a quote by A.A. Milne: "Remember, you are braver than you believe, stronger than you seem, and faster than you think." This quote resonated with me, reminding me that I am tougher and stronger than I believe. This journal has become a vital part of my journey, telling my story from one chapter to the next.

Over the past few years, I became a regular listener of several podcasts about running and nutrition. My favorites were (and still are) *Ali on the Run, Diz Runs, C Tolle Run, Mind Pump, Rambling Runner,* and *Not Your Average Runner.* I first got into podcasts after discovering the extensive world of shows discussing all things running (trail and road), often featuring people like me.

While I enjoyed interviews with running greats like Des Linden, Keira D'Amato, Kara Goucher, and Shalane Flanagan, I preferred listening to the stories of 'regular' runners who shared their triumphs and successes. I heard about runners who continued running through cancer treatment and those who found solace in running while grieving. I listened to podcasts in doctors' waiting rooms and on planes between Newark, New Jersey, and Tel Aviv, Israel.

I joined some podcast groups on Facebook and became a regular poster myself. I had my own 'story' of how I got into running, but I didn't think it was anything special, so I hesitated to respond to the request from *Diz Runs* podcast host, Denny Krahe, to share my running journal on his show. However, I noticed more people from the Facebook group were being featured, so I decided to share my tale. I figured maybe one person would hear my story and relate, just as I had been inspired by many of his followers.

Denny made me feel comfortable from the start of our interview. He asked how I got into running and working out, and it felt more like a conversation than an interview. We discussed my newfound love of trail running, my first Spartan race, and how I transitioned from being a couch potato to embracing fitness.

Talking to Denny on his podcast allowed me to step out of my comfort zone, share my story, and take pride in my accomplishments, whether ringing the bell after finishing an obstacle at the Spartan race or running my first 5K.

I never knew until Jeff told me during a run in early November that I have a certain look when I'm nervous or about to freak out. We met in Brecksville, and he had a plan while I was totally in the dark but eager to follow his lead. I was running fasted, meaning I hadn't eaten or drunk anything since dinner the night before. We maintained a steady pace for the first mile, enjoying the beautiful weather and our easy conversation.

We turned onto a street that led us to the Oak Grove Trails. As I jogged up a seemingly endless hill, I refused to panic or let my guard down. I was determined to reach the top without walking. I focused on the word *FOCUS*, using it as my mantra. I concentrated on my steps forward and upward, continuing without worrying about my speed. It wasn't a race; it was a challenge I was ready to face. I kept my mind on how great I would feel reaching the top before turning around to come back down.

Remember how I was in the dark about Jeff's plan? Well, he had us go right back up that hill a second time, all the way to the top and then back down to the main road. I heard his cues and told myself to 'just do it,' resisting the urge to think it was too hard. I visualized the word *FOCUS* in bright yellow letters. Though I didn't see it, I pictured it in my mind, and it encouraged me. I felt amazing reaching the top, even as my legs started to weaken. I somehow found extra focus to finish the last half mile with as much speed as I could muster.

As for that look I supposedly had, Jeff noticed it after we finished the hill portion and were heading back to the bridge where we parked. With about a mile left for some speed work, we increased our pace every quarter mile. I was just trying to control my breathing, but I guess I looked antsy because Jeff told me to 'get rid of that look.' I knew we still had some running left to do and felt

I needed to hold back a bit, but I also felt close to the end and knew I could finish strong. And I did, giving it everything I had.

A week later, Jeff and I met for the same run. Instead of turning around after what turned out to be the first of several hills, he had me go up for more until we reached a higher point on the road.

As I ran up, I looked ahead at the hills and didn't feel that panicky feeling I'd experienced before. I faced the hills and just ran toward them. I wasn't afraid and didn't worry about how I'd manage to run up those hills. I just did it.

A few weeks later, while driving to meet Jeff for a run in Brecksville, I saw the words "just do it" on a sports car that passed me on the highway. I wasn't sure if it was fate, but they were the perfect words to pump me up for the 10K we were about to do. I had worked hard for this run, and even though I still found the hills leading to the Carriage Trail intimidating, I was determined to tackle them.

I was a few yards from the bridge parking lot when I saw a sign reading "bridge closed ahead." When Jeff arrived, I told him the bridge to the towpath was closed for construction, so we would need another route. He came up with Plan B—running the same course as last week by the Oak Grove hills and then going a little higher for more mileage. Having run this road twice before, I didn't panic when I saw the hills, nor did I flinch when Jeff mentioned we had another big hill to climb. He frequently reminded me to follow him and not push to the front of our line since we were on a winding road.

Finally reaching the road where we turned around was a relief as it was downhill from there. We encountered a few small hills, but since we could run faster downhill, I transitioned better and continued onward. I felt something radiating in my left leg and mentioned it—not to elicit sympathy, but to acknowledge my discomfort while pushing through. I knew the hardest part was behind me, and we had a mile of flat running once we reached the bottom of the road.

On the way back, I said something too loudly like, "I have to stop." It was a moment of weakness, but I didn't mean it; I knew I couldn't stop short. Once again, that mental voice telling me I couldn't do something hard tried to undermine me. Jeff coached me firmly, saying there was no quitting and to silence that voice because I could do this. I reminded myself of the phrase I saw on the car earlier that morning: Just do it.

With a final quarter mile to go, I dashed for the parking lot, just as I had run to the finish the previous weeks. Another strong finish.

On November 26, Jeff and I finally ran the 10K we had talked about for weeks but hadn't been able to do until then. It didn't matter that it was raining all morning and that the trails would be muddy and slippery. I knew I would get wet, and I was okay with that. I wasn't going to overthink getting up the steep hills connecting the towpath to the trails. I was committed to this run no matter what. I layered up and kept my rain jacket on since it was 47 degrees and raining.

I didn't push too fast on the pavement and handled the hills well, facing a climb not as steep as the Carriage Trail. We reached the top and ran across the trails, being careful to avoid sticks, mud, and anything in our way. I never looked at my watch, unaware of the mile markers or our pace. It was all about staying strong and focused, keeping my mind from wandering to negativity.

I felt much better once we were running downhill, knowing we'd soon be back on the towpath with about two miles left. I was feeling spent, but stopping wasn't an option. I struggled not to voice how I couldn't do this anymore, knowing I could finish. Or did I?! We were over a mile from the end when I stopped my watch, and Jeff gave me a well-deserved talking-to! He told me I could handle this and would finish.

I didn't restart my watch but got my feet moving right away, even if it was more of a jog than a run. We passed the parking lot where we had parked our cars since we still had another third of a mile to complete the 10K. Once we turned around to finish, I found a bit more energy and finished strong again. Through the muddy, slippery trails and towpath, I made the impossible a reality. I knew it would be hard and that I'd be running in the rain, but I was determined. And I did!

In December, Gary and I officially became Israeli citizens, allowing us to travel in and out of Israel during the pandemic without issue. I was increasingly frustrated by the few pounds I had gained over the past year, though I knew the cause. In Israel, we relied more on restaurant deliveries and takeout rather than my home-cooked 'cleaner' food.

I decided to follow Jeff's suggestion of a calorie cut to kickstart weight loss while allowing my body to become a fat-burning machine. For 10 days, I restricted my intake to 1,500 calories. Some days, I wasn't fully satisfied with my meals, but I realized I could eat fewer calories than 'normal' to maximize fat loss while maintaining muscle mass. My runs were less intense and easier-paced to support my calorie-cutting efforts. My training sessions still focused on total body workouts, building muscle, and burning fat.

Once I was back in Cleveland, I met Jeff for a measurement assessment (I lost inches thanks to the calorie cut!) and ran a fasted 5K in 29:07 at 39 degrees!

In 2020, I discovered my love for trail running and conquered my fear of hills! I realized that running uphill was as much a mental challenge as a physical one, and it took considerable effort to overcome my fears. I used to avoid any incline during my outdoor runs, opting for flat or downhill routes.

Finally, I began choosing paths that required me to run uphill instead of downhill. My goal for 2021 was to address the mental barriers—the 'I'm afraid,' the 'I can't,' and the 'it hurts.' For too long, I hadn't trusted myself to push beyond my limits mentally, which held me back physically. I understood it was all in my mind. I had completed three half marathons, yet I couldn't imagine running a fourth because it felt like 'too much.' I needed to work on trusting myself and my abilities.

CHAPTER 7

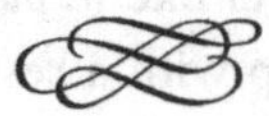

FINISH STRONG

I started 2021 with a speed interval run—but it wasn't just any ordinary run. I was on one treadmill at the gym while my older son, Seth, ran beside me, and my younger son, Yonatan, worked out a few feet away. The idea of working out—better yet, *running*—surrounded by my boys was something I had never pictured for myself.

Two days after that special experience, I went out for a 5K run, feeling uninspired. I had been fasting for 14 hours, but I didn't feel overtired—just indifferent. I would've rather not been doing it, but I told myself to push through. I walked for about ten minutes, then played some fast-paced running music to help motivate me. I intentionally started on an uphill street to get in some hill work, knowing the rest of the route would be flat or downhill.

I tackled the hill the same way I had when I ran with Jeff back in November—moving steadily without racing until I reached the top—then kept going. I didn't check my watch until something nudged me to, and I saw I had already hit three miles. I kept my eye on it until I pressed the stop button at 3.1 miles.

As I walked back to our apartment, I checked my Runkeeper app and saw that my 5K time was 28:04! I was pretty sure I hadn't run a sub-29-minute 5K in two years, so I pulled up my top 5K times. To my surprise, this was my fourth-fastest 5K, and the last time I'd run anything faster was back in July 2017. Three and a half years had passed, and my *second* run of 2021 had me just 1 minute and 22 seconds off my all-time 5K PR.

Reflecting on how I felt at the beginning of that run, I wondered how much faster it could have been had I skipped the hill and stuck to a flat or downhill route. But I chose to embrace the run because I had *started* when I didn't feel like it, *pushed* when it would've been easier to quit, and ended up with a result that genuinely surprised me.

Everything I do—the strength training, the speed intervals, the walking—has made me physically stronger. But the *mental* push is equally important. Building mental strength has taken me to another level. It's what helped turn an uninspired start into a run for the records.

For the first time in a long while, I felt like beating my 5K PR wasn't just possible—it was within reach.

By the end of January, I was back in Cleveland without anything specific to train for—other than my goal of improving my 5K pace. It was too cold to run outside, so I committed to following the same plan I had used for my fifth-fastest 5K a few years back. I started with a 9:30-minute mile pace for the first four minutes—fast for a warm-up, but it felt doable—then alternated one-minute intervals: base pace between 9:05 and 9:22 minutes per mile, and one-minute bursts between 8:06 and 8:34 minutes per mile.

Those bursts were tricky, but I managed to get through each one, feeling motivated and determined to achieve my goal. I hit the 5K mark at 27:44—my fourth-fastest time, just about a minute off my PR. I *could* do this. It felt attainable. It felt very possible.

I joined Strava before January turned into February and participated in a monthly 5K run challenge. It didn't earn me any prizes beyond a virtual badge, but signing up and completing a virtual challenge was more about accountability—and about steadily working toward a goal.

I began another calorie cut, this time aiming for 1,500 calories a day for five days. I got used to the lower calorie count and kept my carbs under 50 grams. I felt satisfied with my meals and didn't miss the side dishes that usually accompanied the main course at dinner.

Gary and I went to Florida for a few weeks to visit our parents and enjoy the warmer weather. While running outside with no pressure to rush or restrict my distance, I found myself stopping short after two miles. I knew I could do more—especially after running distances between 5K and five miles in recent weeks—but running for just 16 or 18 minutes felt inadequate. I felt guilty for doing less, so much so that I didn't share my runs on my MRTT group page as I usually did. I realized something wasn't right, so I told Jeff I felt like I was losing my running mojo again. I was determined to get it back, but I wasn't sure how I had lost it—or how I could reclaim it.

Jeff suggested I enjoy some easy runs. I wasn't exactly sure what that meant, other than running for the pure joy of it, without feeling like I was training for something. My next run was outside in my in-laws' golf community, and I followed Jeff's advice. I left their house and did a run/walk interval: five minutes walking, two minutes running. I took pictures of my surroundings—the houses and greenery—and thought about how fortunate I was to be outside and moving, appreciating that I *got* to do this rather than *had* to do this. I greeted other people walking and jogging and waved to those riding in golf carts. I never could have done any of this on a run focused on finishing in a certain time or pushing for a specific distance. I realized that some runs are meant for pushing and competing, while others serve to remind me how lucky I am to run.

As someone who used to have a cold weather tolerance maximum of 45 degrees, I never thought I would run outside in February—at least not in Cleveland! And as someone who discovered trail running only two years prior and embraced it from the start, I never imagined I'd return to the trails in Cleveland at this time of year. We'd had a lot of snow in the past few months, and the trails were covered in ice and snow—so why would I even *consider* running in such conditions, let alone before warmer temperatures arrived in April?

When Jeff suggested we meet for our first trail run of 2021, I thought, *You want me to do what?!* He assured me it wouldn't be dangerous, but warned that it would be a tough run since I was on day two of a three-day calorie cut and we were increasing activity intensity. My glutes were already sore when I got up, so I did all kinds of stretching to activate them.

We started the run by walking through a field before entering the trails, which were covered in snow, ice, and slush. Jeff cautioned me to stay aware of the ground, since the usual terrain was now hidden. I had to move carefully, especially on the downhills, following his lead by going sideways to stop myself if I slipped. I took my time on the stairs leading to a new trail, deliberately stepping around patches of ice to avoid falling. My glutes were on fire for most of the run—but it was all good.

It was a beautiful experience—slush and all—running through the woods and open fields, hearing laughter from children sledding nearby, and passing several people walking the same trails. I took everything in and appreciated the chance to be outside, no matter how cold it was. We ended the 3.81-mile run with me staying upright the entire time!

My running mojo once again took a roller coaster ride during the spring months of 2021. In March, I went for a run, and everything about it was perfect. I had planned my route and stuck to it, keeping my watch covered with my running jacket sleeve to avoid checking my pace. I ran without concern for time or distance, focusing instead on the joy of running outside in Jerusalem, where ancient and modern times connect. I absorbed my surroundings and felt a tremendous sense of gratitude for the opportunity to run.

However, a week later, I felt anything but grateful. Back in Cleveland, I went for a run without a set time, pace, or distance. My sole intention was to enjoy it—but by half a mile in, I found myself glancing at my watch, willing myself to finish. I sensed a kind of runner's block, if that even exists. I took Jeff's advice and wrote a blog post about my feelings:

> "I love running. I want to run—not just for the physical benefits, but for the mental gains of putting everything on hold and just moving. I see others

running outside and feel wistful, wishing to join them. I gain so much from being part of a Sunday morning group and the Facebook running communities, whether reading Garmin posts or hearing how others get it done.

I have many motivators in my 'real life' and online life, but I feel like I'm suffering from something akin to runner's block. Maybe it's because I haven't raced since February 2020, or because I haven't had anything to train for. I don't understand why I can only manage two miles like I did today.

I love running. I feel a high when I finish, and no matter how I felt at the start, I'm glad I did it. I cherish the sense of accomplishment when I cross a finish line and feel empowered. I've been told I inspire others with my running, but on days like today, I feel anything but inspiring."

I started brainstorming ways to lift myself out of this funk. Should I listen to music instead of a podcast? Run with someone else to avoid boredom?

On April 12, I ran the Towpath Trilogy 5-mile race with Kimi. It was her daughter Rachel's first race—she started with us, then ran ahead and earned a third-place finish in her age group! Kimi and I had planned to enjoy the experience and walk when needed. I was dealing with GI issues that morning, so I wasn't feeling my best, but I still wanted to run with Kimi. We ran a good portion of the race, though I found myself asking to walk during the last two miles.

It felt great to be around people again, soaking in the excitement as we waited for our wave to start. We greeted every volunteer and stopped at the water stations. Kimi hoped to finish in around an hour, and we crossed the line in 1:01:12. I especially loved hearing her tell Rachel how to approach the next race—I think I created a monster!

In late April, I did a trail run with Jeff that reignited the rush of excitement I hadn't felt in a while. On the drive back, I reflected on that post-run high—Jeff had called to check in, and I told him I felt invigorated and energized, and I meant it. After missing two weeks of trail running, we met up at a Cuyahoga Valley National Park trail. I tried not to think about the mileage or the terrain. Bundled up for the thirty-degree weather, I focused on enjoying the run.

We didn't push hard, but it felt challenging enough—and I didn't check my watch once. The rush hit when we finished, despite a moment of doubt as I ran across a grassy hill toward the parking lot. I muttered, "I'm done," but I knew I had to finish the last 50 yards. Out of gas, I pushed myself up the hill with Jeff's encouragement and sprinted to my car.

I wondered whether the rush came from missing the trails or from knowing trail running gives me something nothing else does. I won't assume I'm back to the runner I was in February 2020—before what I now call 'runner's block'—but this run gave me a much-needed boost. It reminded me that the joy, the excitement, and the rush can come from a slow, muddy twelve-minute mile on the trails just as much as from a 10K PR on the streets of downtown Cleveland.

Since my grandchildren were born in April 2020, I had dreamed of taking one—or both—on a run. I hadn't bought a jogging stroller yet, but the intention was always there. That dream finally came true one April Sunday morning during the JCC Stroller 5K with my granddaughter, Arielle. I had originally planned to take her and her twin brother, Ezra, in their double stroller, but he stayed behind for some reason (oh, those toddlers!).

Since I had already run 3.3 miles in Aurora earlier that morning, I decided to walk the 5K—but still, the dream was happening. It was cold outside, but I bundled Arielle up and settled her into the stroller with a cookie as we navigated the course through the JCC parking lot and around the campus three times. Arielle was a trooper, 'chatting' with me occasionally before falling asleep around mile two. I walked briskly, including a few brief running intervals with the stroller, eager to finish and get her out of the cold. She woke just as I completed the 3.1 miles, giving me a big smile as if she had crossed the finish line herself!

The word *awareness* became central to my running vocabulary. Jeff and I met at Hampton Hills on April 28 for our weekly trail run in Cuyahoga Valley National Park. The run flew by, with Jeff leading as we navigated trails that combined typical terrain with the usual lumps and roots we had to avoid. A refreshing breeze cut through the humidity in the open field, and I focused intently on staying aware—whether avoiding debris on the trail or keeping my balance on the hills.

I carried that awareness with me on the drive home, taking in the scenery and wishing I could somehow capture the stunning layers of green and yellow in the trees. I noticed bluish tones in the rocks and even hints of purple and maroon. I felt a deep sense of gratitude—for the run, the stillness, and the awareness it gave me.

I wish I had that same sense of awareness when I went to Brecksville for a solo run on the main road path. I had everything going for me—great weather, beautiful scenery, and a relatively empty path, which was rare considering how many joggers, runners, and walkers are usually out on any given day. I ran easily from the Nature Center parking lot to the bridge parking lot, then turned around to head back.

About six-tenths of a mile from the parking lot, I started to feel a tug in my right hip. I told myself to slow down—I just needed to finish. I began a mental conversation, thankfully unheard by anyone else. *There's that first hill, looking so arrogant, but I'm going to show it I can conquer it.* I slowed as I approached and trotted to the top, feeling victorious. I reassured myself I was strong as I reached the top, caught my breath, and kept going.

I ran toward the second hill, which seemed less daunting, and trotted up. The tugging in my hip returned. *Should I stop? No, don't stop... you're almost there. One more hill to go, but you're not done. But I'm tired and uncomfortable. You can do it... just slow down, but keep going. You're so close.*

I glanced at my watch: three miles. The hardest hill was still ahead. I wavered between *I can do it* and *I've had enough.* At 3.1 miles, I hit the stop button and shifted to a walk to cool down.

Why did I stop? Why didn't I just tackle that last hill?

I mentally berated myself for stopping, knowing I could have continued—even at a slower pace. I had planned to give this run my all, but instead, I gave 98%. Sure, I completed a 5K solo, driving thirty minutes to a beautiful park that offered so much more than my neighborhood. But I let my mind take control and convince me I couldn't reach my full potential.

It was something I needed to work on.

In early May, I decided to make a fresh start. I was supposed to meet Jeff in Peninsula for a trail run, but he was short on time, so we met in Rocky River instead. We began on the pavement, and I immediately felt a sense of familiarity—it was the same path we had run during my first visit to Rocky River four years earlier. It had snowed that day, and I was excited to run through the trails and enjoy the landscape of forests, streams, and ponds.

Fast forward to this run: we maintained a comfortable, chat-worthy pace, though there were moments when Jeff reminded me to control my breathing—and I realized I needed to do just that. The colors of the leaves and bushes were vivid, especially the shades of green that ranged from deep forest to bright lime. I remembered the field that led us from the parkway to the trails, the Nature Center, and the hill we'd walked up in previous runs—one I had never felt brave enough to run. As we passed it, I thought I heard Jeff say, "Let's try it." I didn't mind attempting it now; I knew I could handle hills better than before.

I was determined to complete the run without falling into the mental struggle I had been battling—the voice that told me I was too tired to finish. As we returned to the pavement and neared our starting point, Jeff gave me distance cues: a mile and a quarter, three-quarters of a mile, four-tenths of a mile. I told him I was going to finish this run without mentally or physically bonking out. I felt a tug in my left hip but didn't mention it to Jeff. Instead, I told myself to ignore it. I quickened my pace as we approached the parking lot and ran all the way to my car, completing our 4.74-mile run. I felt stronger than I had on previous runs—likely because I stayed focused and didn't let my mind drift into negative self-talk. Could this be the beginning of my fresh start?

I also followed up on Jeff's suggestion to try destination running to help break through my on-and-off mental struggles. I already knew that running in my neighborhood didn't inspire me the way trail runs with Jeff, Sunday runs with the Aurora group, or outings with my friend Caroline did. I figured that if I took the time and effort to drive somewhere, I wouldn't stop at two miles. I'd commit to more than 20 minutes and hopefully enjoy the experience more.

I planned to revisit the route I had taken in April—the one where I'd stopped short of running the final hill. That run had left me frustrated and disappointed, not because of the pace or distance, but because I'd given in to the "I can't do this anymore" voice in my head. I had invalidated the effort I put in that day because I didn't finish strong.

This time, I committed to the same route but promised myself I'd take it at an easy pace and conquer every hill on the way back. I was alone in a place that had become familiar—but in truth, I wasn't really alone. As I ran, I passed people walking their dogs, jogging, and running along the same path, smiling and greeting me with a "good morning." It felt good to be out there, enjoying the trail without feeling rushed or pressured to finish quickly.

I maintained a comfortable pace—it felt more like a jog—and moved along while listening to a podcast and staying aware of my surroundings. I was determined to finish the run without stopping, and sure enough, I saw 3.22 miles on my watch when I returned to the starting point 35 minutes later. In my last run on that route, I'd finished 3.1 miles at a pace 30 to 35 seconds faster than today's. But this run was better—because I took my time. The quality of the run mattered more than the quantity.

I've learned that good intentions don't always lead to the best results. I've made many mistakes along this journey—ones I wish I could undo. Going to the bathroom after mile 2 during a mile repeat run at Acacia? Big mistake. Running the day after a 10K or half marathon? Another big mistake.

I had the best intentions the day before a big trail run with Jeff. I took an easy two-mile walk before our virtual training session and another two-mile walk afterward. I hydrated with water and unsweetened iced tea that morning and didn't push the pace of either walk, especially given the heat at 10:30. But I didn't hydrate enough in the hours after—and I paid the price.

The morning of our trail run, I woke up with a bad headache and some GI issues. I told Jeff I wasn't feeling my best but insisted

I'd be fine to run. I took some Motrin for the headache, and after an hour and a half, I felt better. But about an hour before we were supposed to meet, Jeff called and suggested I skip the run. And then came the talk.

I may have had good intentions with those walks the day before, but I hadn't considered how hot and humid it was—or how poorly I had planned for hydration afterward. The run we had scheduled was meant to be one of the most challenging I'd ever do… if not *the* most challenging. It would've been great practice for our upcoming Spartan race. The walks didn't tire me out, but not hydrating properly before and after was a huge mistake. Deep down, I knew I'd messed up.

Too often, I get so caught up in staying active and pushing myself that I don't fully consider the consequences of what *seems* like the right thing. Running solo on a hilly path two days before a demanding trail run? That can strain my calf. Running on a day when I've been traveling? That can wreak havoc on my body. Overdoing it or overtraining leads to overuse injuries—and I've learned the hard way that it's not worth getting sidelined because I did too much, instead of doing less and feeling good afterward.

There are still days when I think that if I run more or stay extra active—especially on days I shouldn't—I'll see the inches melt away or the pounds drop. But this conversation with Jeff made me realize I'm still clinging to an old mindset: that the numbers on the scale or the measuring tape matter more than doing the right thing for my body.

Two days later, I tackled that challenging trail run with Jeff. The forecast called for rain, and I quickly accepted that I would get wet—and that was okay. As I drove out to meet Jeff for the Butlers Trail run, I told myself I would embrace getting wet, just as I had embraced wading through muddy waters during my first Spartan race.

We started with a half-mile run along the road before heading to Butlers Trail, located on the opposite side of the road from our previous run. It was raining, but not heavily on the road, and it seemed light as we ran through the trails. There were many steep hills; I ran some but had to walk more than I would have liked. It was muddy and wet, and I enjoyed every minute of it—even crossing streams without anything to step on to avoid going feet-first into the water. I got wet, and you know what? I didn't care! My shoes were soaked, my socks were soggy, and I was pretty sure my pants were splattered with mud. But honestly, I didn't care.

Well... maybe I cared a little when I noticed my "quick-dry" shirt was anything but dry, and I made a mental note to ask Amazon for a partial refund.

After one trail, Jeff announced we had run 1.6 miles, and I could have sworn we had gone much farther. We kept going, with just under three miles left. This run challenged me—with the hills we climbed and descended—but I never felt the urge to stop. At one point, we looked up at a hill we had just run up and across, and I couldn't believe I had actually done that.

When we finally emerged from the trails and reached the main road, I was definitely winded—but I still found the strength to sprint to my car and finish strong.

On June 7, I participated in my second Spartan Sprint with Jeff and one of my Aurora running friends, Nicole. Jeff and I had registered as a team back in 2019, and we all know how the May 2020 race was postponed and then canceled. Fortunately, we were able to use our entries for the next Midwest Sprint, held in Garrettsville, Ohio (just a 45-minute drive from my house).

During one of my runs with the Aurora group, I mentioned I'd be doing a Spartan race, and Nicole asked if she could join our team. Why not?! That was the name of our team, and Jeff and I were more than happy to include her and add her talents to the experience.

This Spartan was a completely different beast than my first. The trails were super muddy—I was convinced a fleet of trucks had dumped mud all over them just before race weekend. It wasn't easy running through the mud; I slipped once in the woods, dirtying my capris and thighs in the process. The slick conditions made the obstacles even harder, especially right after emerging from the trails.

I attempted as many obstacles as I could—I scaled the four-foot wall twice with a little boost from Jeff, and I completed all the heavy carries, including holding a 100-pound metal ball while walking back and forth. I carried a cooler filled with rocks up and down hills, and slung a sandbag across my neck and shoulders as I hiked up and down inclines. And of course, I did the Hercules Hoist —my favorite obstacle from my first Spartan—pulling a heavy weight to the top of the rig and lowering it slowly, without letting it slip.

There were a few obstacles I knew I wouldn't attempt—the monkey bars and the rope climb—but fortunately, my teammates aced most of them. I navigated the scaling wall, where we had to move across the outside edge with minimal footing and grip. I took my time and made it through. I also tackled the super high A-frame tower, climbing up one side and switching over to descend the other. That one was tough for me, since I've always been afraid of heights, and the structure shook from the movement of fellow Spartans as I climbed.

I crawled under the barbed wire, keeping my body low, and eventually resorted to rolling for the final stretch. There was one obstacle I had trained for—the slanted wall that had pushed me mentally and physically two years ago—but with my shoes caked in mud, I didn't feel confident. I felt bad skipping it, but I knew it would've been too much in that moment.

The three of us ended up doing five rounds of burpees, which we split among us, all in good spirits and fun. I was on such a high from the experience that my head was in the clouds as we ran over the fire pit—and instead of leaping over it, I stepped right into it! I felt the flames lick my right calf as the clock read 1:33:18.

The high I felt came from being part of an experience, not just a race. The other participants were so friendly—it didn't feel like a competition at all. Racers helped each other over obstacles and cheered each other on. The burn on my thigh would fade and eventually disappear, but the memories of this Spartan race would stay with me for a long time.

My fitness journey has always revolved around goal setting. It all started with a simple goal—to run. Six years later, I had completed countless 5Ks, 10Ks, half marathons, trail races, and two

Spartan Sprints. Every time I finished a big race or wrapped up a training block, Jeff would tell me it was time to set a new goal.

I've set goals to improve my pace and increase my distance, but each time I needed to come up with something new, I'd find myself stumped. The day after my second Spartan race, I talked with Jeff about what my next goal should be—and asked him what he thought it should be too.

I admitted that I wanted to start practicing daily mindfulness. Just a few minutes a day of intentional stillness—stretching, breathing, and letting go. I tend to stress and overthink, especially about things I can't control, and I wanted to make a real effort to change that. It sounded simple and totally doable.

But all that Zen went right out the window when Jeff told me his goals for me: to run a 10K trail race that summer *and* clock my fastest 5K ever. I told him I was up for both—but they'd have to wait until I returned from Israel in late July. My son and his wife were expecting a baby boy in early July, and I wanted to be fully present for that moment. After that? I was ready to take on whatever training plan Jeff came up with.

I was determined to beat my 5K PR, but I will admit I freaked out when Jeff set the goal at 25 minutes. My fastest 5K was 26:48, so shaving off a minute and 48 seconds would take a lot of effort. I was game—nervous, excited, and ready. I loved having a specific schedule for the time I was away and something to train for.

The training plan called for running four days a week and virtual training sessions twice a week, focusing on building strength. The runs included an easy run on Sunday, where I would keep the pace easy but increase the distance each week; a speed interval run on Monday, where I would push the sprint pace and time; a mile repeat run on Wednesday, where I would run faster paces for a mile at a time—much faster than any mile repeat pace I had done in previous training plans; and on Friday, I would dedicate myself to running a 5K as fast as possible.

I ran a 27:49 5K as a baseline for my PR goal. Each Friday, I pushed myself more and more to beat that baseline time and aim for a 25-minute 5K. I thought beating my 26:48 5K was the goal, but we would be going further and faster over the next six weeks. It all seemed daunting and nearly impossible, but I was determined!

My Friday runs would focus on running as hard and better than I ever had. A 25-minute 5K—could I really do it? I remembered asking myself that same question just before my first 5K race, again at each of my Spartan races, and I was pretty sure I had asked that question every time I participated in any race.

I wouldn't know for sure until I saw that number in front of me, but I was ready to take a leap of faith and say I could really do this!

Once I realized that a 25-minute 5K equated to an 8:03 overall pace, I panicked and asked myself that familiar question: "You want me to do what?!"

I even had a little freak-out after sharing my intentions with friends and family and wondered if I should text Jeff to say I couldn't do this challenge after all. I knew I had put myself out there by sharing this goal because I felt it would make me more accountable, and I realized there was no sense in quitting before I had even started. I was going to do this.

I ran my first attempt at the 5K challenge on June 18. I did a three-minute warm-up jog to get my legs ready, then started the 5K run at a pace that felt comfortably challenging. I maintained a running pace between 11.2 and 11.3 kilometers (8:32–8:36 minute mile pace) and reached the 5K mark in 26:42. I set a new PR!

I reveled in the moment, given my initial fears and doubts about this task becoming a reality. I hadn't thought I could surpass my previous 26:48 PR, but I did. I hadn't believed I could maintain such a fast pace for more than a few minutes, yet I did just that for over 26 minutes!

The supposedly impossible challenge I had taken on seemed achievable. I just had to believe I could do it.

This training plan was proving more challenging than the half marathon plans I had followed in the past. I had more to accomplish in less time and a specific goal to pursue, rather than just preparing for a half marathon race.

The leap from 26:42 to 25 minutes felt daunting… it all seemed so impossible and unreal, but I knew I had to shift my mindset to embrace the challenge instead of doubting my ability to pull it off.

When I attempted the challenge a week later, I increased my speed to between 11.3 and 11.5 kilometers and finished in 26:17. Having music at 180 bpm helped me stay motivated and focused, but that run was definitely harder than the week before.

The following week, I completed it in 26:15 (an 8:28 minute mile pace!)—two minutes faster than the prior week—and I ran it on a treadmill alongside Yonatan. Initially, I thought that shaving only two seconds wouldn't be good enough for my efforts, but considering I had run side by side with my son and finished strong, I felt it was sufficient.

I practiced mind over matter the following week and finished my 5K in 25:55. I used the same focus I had during my plank for 90 seconds straight after an intense training session. I stared at a spot on the gym floor as Jeff called out the time every 15 seconds and focused on that spot as my legs began to shake, telling myself I could do this.

When I ran the 5K challenge that Friday (two days after my grandson Aidan was born), I increased the pace to 11.6 kilometers and gradually moved it to 11.8 kilometers. I felt the need to hold onto the handles for a few seconds now and then, but I tried my best to run hands-free at that pace.

The higher speed was more than I could handle, and I began to think I should have held back and maintained a lower pace consistently, rather than relying on the handles to help me sustain the faster pace.

The following week, I ran the 5K in 25:31. My training had been going well, and I was running an 8:33 minute mile pace for my mile repeats. For this run, I started the 5K at an 11.6 kilometer pace and maintained it for three minutes before increasing to 11.7 kilometers for another seven minutes, then to 11.8 kilometers for the remainder of the run.

The 11.7 and 11.8 kilometer paces proved difficult for running hands-free, and once again, I found myself grasping the handles for support. Should I have held back on pace and stuck to something more manageable, like 11.5 or 11.6 kilometers, and run that consistently to stay hands-free? I didn't know the answer, but I focused on getting through my training runs, one day at a time, giving them everything I had.

A week later, I ran the 5K in 25:29, meaning I had shaved off nearly a minute and 20 seconds from my original PR during this challenge. I couldn't believe the numbers I had achieved… was this really me—the Hildee who had always tripped over herself and struggled with lunges at the beginning of this fitness journey?!

25:29 was closer to the 25-minute mark—something worth celebrating. I had worked hard on my speed intervals and mile repeats, and I knew they contributed to that time, just as much as the virtual training workouts I had done that week. I refused to let myself feel down for not going faster or not being closer to the 25-minute mark.

I was in the final week of the challenge. After my stretching warm-up, I hopped on the treadmill for a three-minute low-intensity warm-up. I set the pace to an 8:28-minute mile and increased it every 30 seconds for the first two minutes. Then I bumped it up to an 8:11-minute mile for about eight minutes, followed by an 8:07-minute mile for the next ten. I settled into an 8:03-minute mile pace for the remainder of the run—it felt like my ultimate pushing pace.

I approached this run ready to give it everything I had.

I finished in 25:13, averaging an 8:08-minute mile pace overall. I was incredibly proud of that time and pace, especially reflecting on where I started this challenge.

I couldn't ignore the work I'd put in to get there. The mile-repeat runs had me holding paces I'd never managed before, and the speed intervals pushed me with longer bursts and more reps. Strength training had fortified both my upper and lower body, giving me the stability and power to take on those weekly PR challenges.

Each week, I moved closer to a goal that once felt impossible—and even though I didn't quite reach it, I got pretty damn close.

Once upon a time, I made a list of goals for myself, and after coming so close to meeting the 5K PR goal and overcoming my fear of hill running, I moved that list to the trash file on my phone. The third item on that list was to hold a two-minute plank during a virtual training session.

Over the years, I had done a plank or two for more than two minutes and even gotten close to three minutes, but it had been a long time since I managed more than a 30- or 45-second plank in a circuit. For this plank challenge, I started with a one-minute straight arm plank.

Over the following weeks, I increased my plank time by thirty seconds until I reached two and a half minutes. Planking was hard! It required tremendous physical strength and mental focus, and I had to be mindful of my positioning to avoid weakening as time passed and letting that mental monster tell me I couldn't hold on.

I focused on keeping my core tight, my arms straight, and finding something to concentrate on while Jeff counted off every 15 seconds. I completed two separate two-and-a-half-minute planks and thought I could check that goal off my list.

But then Jeff suggested I go for a three-minute plank. Whether it was a moment of pure insanity or a moment of "why not," I agreed to the challenge—but told him he would have to do a plank too.

There we were—he on the floor in his basement, and I on the floor in mine—and we held that straight arm plank for three minutes. Challenge completed!

Two days after completing the 5K PR challenge, I went out for an easy run, considering it a reward for my accomplishment. I ran with the sole intention of moving my legs and ignoring the watch on my left wrist. This run wasn't about duration or speed; it was purely about running until I felt done—without being 'done in.'

It was sunny and in the 70s when I started at 7:45 AM, and I had plenty of time to cover a few miles. I took in the sights and was fully aware of my surroundings, hearing and seeing everything as I ran mostly on pavement through my neighborhood.

I especially enjoyed descending the hill leading to the walls of Jerusalem's Old City and then climbing back up to the modern section of the city. I made my way onto the city running path, passing parents walking their children to school, and admired an elderly man dancing to some music.

I kept going, knowing I had more energy, but reminded myself not to speed up and to run according to feel. I was aware that I had lost that sense of urgency over the past year and several months. I used to love running every time I stepped outside or crossed the finish line, but that excitement had faded.

I wondered if it was because I hadn't had any races to train for and had relied more on treadmills than on roads and trails. Whatever the reason, I had lost my motivation for running and had learned to accept being slower—not running as hard as I did at the beginning of my journey.

I knew I could do more—that I could run beyond the three miles that had become my norm and see an eight or nine in the minutes-per-mile. The 5K challenge reignited that spark. I had something to work for, and each run was done with intention and focus.

While I didn't reach the official goal of a 25-minute 5K, I shaved a minute and 29 seconds off my previous personal record, which felt like a win. I set out on this easy run excited because I could run without worrying about the numbers on my watch. I enjoyed the scenery and knew this was something I could do, not something I had to do.

On August 8, I ran the Hofbrau 10K with Kimi. She aimed for an hour and twenty minutes, and I was confident we could finish in less—even if we had to walk a bit.

It was 75 degrees when we started, and we ran as much as we could before switching to a fast walk occasionally. We stopped at each water station, thanking the police officers managing traffic at various intersections along the course.

I felt the heat, but I enjoyed the experience of running with my friend, who embraced the sport with enthusiasm and joy, and shared our gratitude for being able to move! I had missed the racing experience. I couldn't recall how many races I used to run each year before Covid hit and events were canceled or switched to virtual.

I longed to participate again, and it had been a while since I felt that excitement when I registered for a race and picked up my packet. I had forgotten what it felt like to be nervous and excited on race morning. I even missed the bathroom lines, but on this race day, I remembered it all!

As for Kimi's time goal? We finished in 1:09:43!

Even though the 25-minute 5K PR challenge was over in July, I wasn't done with the competitive side of things. I had come so close to that 25-minute mark and was thrilled with my result of 25:13, but then Jeff announced that we would run a 5K together in Brecksville once I returned to Cleveland in August—and I would be pushing for that goal again.

The panic and sense of *uh-oh* returned, but I tried not to dwell on negative *I can't* thoughts. Instead, I focused on how I would achieve this. That 24:59 number seemed to taunt me, feeling out of reach despite my near success with 25:13. I resolved to go for it and push myself to run hard.

I knew I couldn't let anything get in my way—not the predicted storms nor the fact that I had been awake since 3 AM that morning. I drove to Brecksville, where the forecast called for 75 degrees and humidity at our 7 AM meetup. I took a few deep breaths, reminding myself that I would see this through.

Jeff and I met in the parking lot, warmed up, and walked to our starting point. He agreed to track our run on his watch so I wouldn't be distracted by checking the time and pace. Once we crossed the bridge and Jeff took a few pictures of the beautiful scenery, we took off.

I led the way, and Jeff told me I was pushing a seven-minute pace. I held back, settling into a sustainable rhythm while tuning into my breathing—pushing hard but not gasping for air. We crossed the Station Road Bridge and continued onto the towpath, staying on it for about a mile before turning around.

There were times my breathing intensified, but I tried to regain control without slowing my pace. It was hot and humid, but I didn't let it hinder me.

With a mile left, Jeff guided me through the distance until we reached the finish. He pressed the stop button on his watch, and I asked for our time. He said, "29:17." He was happy and excited, giving me a high five, but I wondered, *what about that sub-25 minute 5K?* He laughed and said it was never about the number.

Okay, so all those weeks of mile repeats, speed intervals, and Friday 5K challenge runs definitely counted! Each run during that training period taught me to push hard and go beyond my comfort zone, both physically and mentally. I ran 5Ks in the 25- and 26-minute range, and each PR was a step toward a goal.

While I didn't reach that 25:00 mark, I got close enough to remind myself that I can do hard things and not let the *I can'ts* hold me back.

Was I disappointed in our run that morning? No way. I gave it my best effort and have no regrets. What began as a run focused on a number turned into a test of myself.

I suddenly found myself without a plan. I still had my two training days a week with Jeff but nothing specific to follow on my running days. I found I actually liked that. I could run with friends without focusing on pace, enjoying the company of Caroline or Kimi. I could go on solo runs and choose my route without worrying about how many miles I could cover in X minutes.

I felt my mojo returning, having just trained for my 5K PR, but this newfound flexibility brought back the joy that had been missing for too long.

Getting out of my comfort zone was something I continued to work on. I began my fitness journey seven years ago as someone uncoordinated who hid behind baggy tops and leggings. Today, I wear fitted tops and compression bottoms, and I'm not afraid of being photographed during a run.

One Wednesday morning in late August, I met Jeff at the Rocky River Nature Center for a quick run and outdoor circuit workout. It was hot, so I wore a tank top and capris. I didn't worry about whether my top made me look top-heavy or if my bottom was sticking out too much. Not a single negative thought crossed my mind as Jeff and I ran through the trails, taking in the view of a beautiful stream surrounded by a high wall that seemed to date back to the dinosaur era. I was sweaty with wet marks on my top, feeling freer than I had in a long time.

After our run, Jeff and I set up for our circuit workout by a picnic area. We had worked out there before, and it was on the grassy corner across from the Nature Center parking lot, with many people walking by and cars passing. I focused on my moves and form rather than worrying about what others might think.

One man complimented us on our workout, and we chatted briefly. I shared how I had been working with Jeff for over seven years and how he helped transform my life. In that moment, I felt completely comfortable sharing my journey—from being sedentary and uncoordinated to running road and trail races and completing two Spartans.

Talking about myself with a stranger pushed me out of my comfort zone. Agreeing to work out in a public setting pushed me out of my comfort zone. Allowing Jeff to take pictures of me working out for his new coaching business pushed me out of my comfort zone.

Jeff had warned me that the Full Moon 4-mile trail race would be tough, and it was! On August 25, I drove to Brecksville by the Oak Grove Reservation with only one expectation: to finish. I hadn't previewed the course, and the temperature was in the mid-90s.

I knew the race sponsors wouldn't call me to tell me to turn around, and I was somewhat conditioned for the heat since I had run in similar conditions with Jeff the year before. I hydrated earlier in the day and completed my stretching routine in the parking lot while waiting for the race to start. I felt prepared.

I didn't have the queasy stomach I usually experience before a race, nor did I feel the last-minute nerves that often accompany lining up at the starting line. The bell rang, and off we went.

I ran this race solo—well, as solo as you can with about 200 participants. Jeff was running his own race, and I was fine with that. I kept a steady pace, watching for debris on the ground and jumping from rock to rock as we crossed a few streams.

I walked several times on the steep hills, but it seemed everyone else was doing the same. It wasn't that I was afraid to run the hills; I had grown more comfortable with it. However, given the heat and the race's length, I knew better than to risk depleting my energy.

Running on my own, I absorbed the new trails and surroundings. I had run in various parts of Brecksville but had never taken this particular trail before, and I wanted to enjoy it fully. I truly didn't care about my time or pace; I just wanted to finish without getting lost or tripping—fears I had about running on trails alone.

There were signs along the way to guide us, and I was surrounded by people, so I knew I wasn't entirely alone. In the last quarter mile, I sprinted toward the finish line, just as I do at the end of every run with Jeff—finishing strong, proud, and accomplished.

I was on such a high driving home and felt great for about an hour after arriving. But then I saw the news: one of the participants had collapsed near the end. There were no details, only that a fellow runner, who was a nurse, had tended to him before an ambulance arrived.

The next morning, I read on Facebook that the man had passed away. I didn't know him and hadn't been there when he collapsed, but I was devastated. I realized that being able to run is truly a privilege and a blessing. It's something I *get* to do, not just something I *have* to do.

I often approached running as an obligation, feeling negative before a run, but by the end, I was always glad I had done it. 47:39 —I'll take it.

Not having a real plan in September rekindled my love of running (along with a plank PR of three minutes!). I could run on the treadmill, but I chose to run outside as much as possible while the weather was good. I ran for as long as I wanted, without worrying about my pace since I wasn't training for anything yet.

I changed my route as I pleased, without a set plan, just enjoying the outdoors. As I turned 53, I wished for a year of getting fitter, leaner, and stronger—both physically and mentally.

On October 29, I ran a 10K in 1:03:06 on the JCC treadmill despite a twinge in my hip. I kept going, ignoring the discomfort and varying my pace without pushing too hard. I listened to a guided run podcast, passing the five-mile mark and then the five-and-a-half-mile mark. I aimed to reach the 10K distance to beat my previous record time and add miles to my monthly Strava challenge.

While walking through the parking lot to my car, a woman stopped to say how impressed she was with my running and how I just kept going. I blushed, thanked her, and told her it meant a lot since I hadn't felt motivated lately.

On the drive home, I realized I had been feeling stuck with my pace and endurance. I knew I had run farther than a 10K in my earlier running years, and it had seemed effortless back then. I marveled at the paces I achieved on Runkeeper. I acknowledged I was older and things had changed, but I still wanted to run a 10K outside (or on the treadmill) in under an hour and improve my speed on the treadmill.

I wondered if I was in a funk because I hadn't been following a specific plan. I enjoyed running without a plan, but had I held myself back? Was I not challenging myself to step outside my comfort zone?

I knew I had it in me. I could run faster; I just needed a push to revive the runner I used to be.

I started training for the 2022 Jerusalem Marathon 10K at the beginning of November, aiming to beat my PR of 1:07:30. I knew I had a lot of work to do on my pace and hill training, and I was determined to focus on that over the next few months. While I was in Israel for a few weeks, Jeff sent me a detailed training schedule that would take me to March 25!

I had run the 10K twice and was familiar with the course, but I wasn't conditioned for the four very steep hills.

I did a solo hill run at Oak Grove in Brecksville, completing four intervals of an eighth of a mile down the hill and then running back up. Running on pavement up and down the hills was the closest I could get to what I'd need to do in the coming months.

A few weeks later, I went out for a hill run in 31-degree weather, instructed to do six rounds of walking down two-tenths of a mile and then turning right back up. The first round went perfectly, but during the second interval, I felt frostbite in a few fingers, and the cold affected my breathing.

I slowed my pace and ended up walking the last part of the hill to the top. I felt like I had cheated because I hadn't run the entire way up. The same thing happened in the third, fourth, and fifth intervals—I simply didn't have it in me to run. I made it through the sixth round, but still felt like I hadn't executed the run correctly.

Did I give it my all when I ran up each time, even if my paces weren't "sprint that sucker," as Jeff had advised? Yes.

Was the cold a factor in compromising my breathing and endurance? Definitely.

I would like to think that had it not been so cold, I could have handled those hills better without resorting to those brief walking breaks. I knew I could have done hill intervals on the treadmill in the comfort of my basement gym or the JCC, but running on pavement, up and down the hills, was the closest preparation for the race ahead.

Jeff sent me a picture of myself from 2019, "posing" in my workout clothes during one of my monthly assessments at the JCC. I was wearing a tank top and capri pants, standing straight and looking at the camera. My reaction was, "I looked pretty lean... then." I couldn't recall exactly when the picture was taken, but I assume it was before my son got married in December, as I had been working hard to rock my mother-of-the-groom gown.

I could see a waistline and the beginnings of triceps in my upper arms, and I was grinning, wishing Jeff would just take that picture and be done with it. The monthly pictures were meant to capture moments in time and show the progress I had made since the summer of 2014. I found myself wishing I looked as lean as I did then, doubting Jeff's reassurance that I looked just as good, if not better, now.

I knew this was a mental hurdle, and until I could truly believe it, I had to trust Jeff, who had guided me to this point.

Before we started an intense workout focused on strength and deadlifts—one of my weaker skills—I took another look at the picture while waiting in my car to pick up my grandson from school. It hit me: I was stronger at 53 than I was in 2019. I could complete three rounds of 15 chest presses with 15-pound weights and swing a 20-pound kettlebell.

Since that picture was taken, I had participated in two Spartan races and numerous trail runs in Brecksville, Rocky River, and Peninsula with Jeff. I had run in snow, ice, cold rain, and 90-degree heat. All of that made me mentally stronger.

I still couldn't see my body as lean and strong as in that picture, and although my weight had increased, Jeff reminded me that the photo was just a snapshot in time. The image of me at 53 was a wife, mother, and grandmother who could play with her grandchildren and lift them for some bicep work. That was something to take pride in.

On Thanksgiving, I ran my first Turkey Trot. For years, I had seen pictures of my friends' past races and heard their stories. Since I was in Cleveland on Thanksgiving and had no reason not to participate, I signed up for the 5K with my friend Frankie.

As race day approached, I realized I would be in my fourth week of training, and this run would be an "extra" run, as I had specific types of runs planned to prepare for the Jerusalem 10K. My attitude was about having a good time, not about a specific finish time.

My youngest daughter, Liat, who was home from Israel, asked me to sign her up last minute. Despite the forecast of rain and showers, I didn't want to skip a race we could do together. We decided to go for it, even with an 80–90% chance of rain.

So, it was Frankie, Liat, and our friends Miki and Ilanit heading downtown. We donned our running gear, took pictures at the expo, and made our way to the starting line. I told Liat to run her own race since Frankie and I would be slower. Frankie and I started together, but after the first mile and a half, she encouraged me to go ahead.

Without music, I focused on my pace. There were people walking dogs, pushing double strollers, and a family in Thanksgiving costumes. I started with a jog, but after passing the mile 2 marker, I pushed a little harder, determined to run the entire course.

Before I knew it, we passed the old courthouse where Frankie serves as a domestic relations judge, and then I saw the finish line. I finished in 35:06—overall, a fun race experience that gave me a reason to be thankful on what could have been an ordinary Thanksgiving.

In the days following the Turkey Trot, I was sidelined with GI issues and had to take three days off. The thought of resting bothered me; I had become accustomed to being active. I understood the need for rest, but it was still hard.

When I returned to the gym, I started with a jog, aiming for a 5K while gauging how I felt. I began at a 12-minute pace for 10 minutes, then increased the pace for another 10 minutes. It felt comfortable, and I didn't experience any pain.

I pushed the pace again for five-minute intervals, aiming to complete a 5K and go beyond to finish a 40-minute timed run from the previous day's calendar. When I stopped the treadmill at 40 minutes, I felt triumphant: "I'm back!" I hadn't run as fast as I could have, but I got through it, and it felt exhilarating!

As I continued training for the Jerusalem 10K, I set two goals: run the entire course—including four steep hills—and finish in less than an hour and seven minutes.

As November turned into December, I began to worry about the second goal. Setting a time meant I would feel great if I achieved it, but I would feel like a failure if I fell short. I questioned whether I should have set a time goal, knowing it takes time to get through the crowd at the start.

I was overthinking it and couldn't let my fears take over, but I still wondered, "Could I really do this?!" I would certainly try. I needed to shift my focus to how I would feel when I finished—and when I put that medal around my neck.

One day, as I was five minutes into my 50-minute treadmill run, my son, Seth, walked in and got on the treadmill next to me. He ran at a pace I could sustain for only a couple of minutes. We ran side by side, and I realized this was a moment to celebrate.

During the years I raised Seth and his four siblings, I never imagined running alongside any of them—let alone on my own. I hadn't been physically active and had focused on caring for others before considering my own needs. As I jogged next to Seth, I wished I could speed up and show him my potential. But then I realized we were both doing our own thing together—a dream I hadn't clearly seen before, but it was a dream come true.

I felt a bit bad when I came nine kilometers short of the 100-kilometer running distance Strava challenge for December. This was the third time I had joined the challenge, and the second consecutive month I fell short of the mark. I could view this as a failure and beat myself up over it—or I could have added those 9 kilometers in the past week to earn that virtual badge—but I didn't.

I followed the training plan strictly and didn't exceed what each run and workout called for, knowing that overachieving leads to overuse and potential injuries. Would I let that badge define my success or failure as a runner?

Instead, I celebrated having run 91 kilometers in December and finishing the month with an amazing speed interval run that morning. I pushed myself with speed bursts, running at a 7:26-minute mile for each 60-second interval—a personal best. The rush and accomplishment I felt upon finishing were no different than after a race. While I hadn't received a medal for that run, it was okay. I finished the month with a bang.

CHAPTER 8

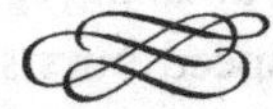

THE 5K THAT CHANGED EVERYTHING

I started 2022 with a side-by-side run with my youngest daughter in the gym at our apartment complex. We each did our own thing on the treadmill: I completed my five-and-a-half-mile long run while she sprinted alongside me. I was so impressed with her—she had taken up running less than two years prior and was already in the mid–eight-minute mile range! This made me reflect on my kids and the memories I have of running and racing with them.

I remember hugging my oldest daughter at the finish line after her first 5K, walking together at another 5K race—unaware she would soon discover she was pregnant—and running my third half marathon with my son, where I set a new PR by 14 seconds. He coached me throughout that race, helping me through tough moments, and I am forever grateful to him for holding back his usual pace to run alongside me and motivate me.

How could I forget emerging from the Old City during my first Jerusalem Marathon 10K to hear, *"Hi Mom!"* My middle daughter was running her first 10K and had been worried about hitting a specific time goal. There she was, greeting me at the halfway point. Seeing her for those few seconds made me feel less alone in my race—even with thousands of other runners around me.

Over the years, I've had a few regular runs with my younger son who, like his older brother, slowed his pace to run with me. Each of those "Mom and me" runs allowed us to bond without interruptions. As for his younger sister, who was sprinting next to me, I was amazed at how seamlessly she has become a runner. I could never take credit for getting my kids into running; each of them pursued it on their own, without any prompting from me. When I started my fitness journey, I hoped to be a role model for my kids—showing them it's never too late to make a change and that hard work pays off.

As I continued training for the 10K that January, I did something I never thought I would do: I signed up for another half marathon.

It all began when I asked my friend Kimi if she wanted to do the Towpath Trilogy 5-miler in April. We had enjoyed the race in 2021, and I thought it would be fun to do it again. Her response? *"Let's do the half marathon."*

"The half?" I asked, unsure if I had heard her correctly.

"I have big dreams," she said.

I had been convinced I would never run another half, but after hearing Kimi's words, I paused to consider what she was really saying. She had started running only two years earlier and always had such a positive attitude. We had completed a few races together during that time, and I enjoyed watching her grow as a runner. Her pace had improved, and she had worked on her distance with an open mind.

I had been sure I was done with half marathons. After three and all the hard training, I didn't want to put in the effort for longer runs. I was focused on training for the 10K in March and looking forward to the rest week afterward. The Towpath half was scheduled for just two and a half weeks after the 10K. Could I really do it?

When I asked Jeff if it was possible, he assured me we could incorporate a half marathon training plan into the one I had been following. Then I thought again about Kimi and her big dreams. What was my real hesitation? How could I say no to running this half marathon with a friend who inspired me?

I wanted to have big dreams like her—to pursue something that seemed just beyond my reach, but achievable with hard work. I wanted to adopt Kimi's open mind and fresh attitude. Before I could change my mind again, I registered for the half and let Kimi know: we were on!

My husband and I spent much of January and February in Florida, where I could run outside and continue my training plan. While running a 5K in my in-laws' golf community, I reflected on my running journey. I was clearly not the same runner I was when I started in 2015. I was older, with less stamina and less of the innocence I once had. While I still derived physical and mental benefits from running, I lacked the drive I once possessed. I knew I couldn't turn back time, but I wished I could be the runner I was in 2016 and 2017.

Occasionally, I would check Runkeeper and feel nostalgic looking at my routes and mile splits from long runs, wishing I could just run those distances again—forget about the paces! I recognized much of this was mental; I wasn't saying I couldn't do it again. I had become trapped in a competitive mindset, which was not a pleasant place to be. I wanted to go for a seven- or eight-mile run without needing to stop midway because I was too tired. I didn't care how fast or slow I ran those miles; I just wanted to be able to do it. I needed to reignite my passion.

Building my self-confidence and mindset had been challenging. Questioning my ability to achieve a goal—and committing to it—was a struggle. Taking on something new, no matter how daunting, was something I had learned to do, but it remained a work in progress. Even with supportive people around me, I couldn't fully trust myself to know what was best. I had lacked confidence for too long to take on running because I was convinced I couldn't do it. Jeff believed in me when I didn't believe in myself and pushed me to start.

Reflecting on how I built confidence over the last few years, it was hard to acknowledge all the things I had accomplished that I once thought were impossible. I ran my first 5K alone, standing at the starting line surrounded by strangers, nervous and questioning whether I should race or turn back. But when the gun went off, I decided to run with them. I followed the other runners, relying on the signs that guided us, and somehow made it through 3.1 miles. A dear friend, who finished well before me, cheered me on as I crossed the finish line—and I will never forget the feeling of achieving the impossible.

I've completed more races alone than with friends, which required confidence. I've tackled 10K and half marathon distances, all of which demanded self-assurance. Trail running opened a new world for me, pushing me to try something vastly different from my previous experiences. Running through mud and climbing five-, six-, or seven-foot walls at a Spartan race—often with my running buddy lifting me—required me to dig deep and find the confidence to prove to myself that I could do it.

Registering for my fourth half marathon, despite being convinced I would never run another, was another test of confidence. Creating my own training plan during the early months of COVID, just to have something to work toward—confidence. Adjusting my training to accommodate an overuse injury, a stubbed toe, or simply needing a rest day—confidence. Gaining confidence meant trusting myself to take on new challenges or make decisions that could be made for me. I had reached a point where I was fully capable of making my own decisions.

Looking back seven years, I could hardly believe that was the same person. I wanted to be someone who could trust herself completely—to go with the flow without doubt or worry. My blog —*You Want Me To Do What?!*—has always been about my fitness journey and doing things outside my comfort zone.

While dealing with Achilles pain in my heel, I learned the importance of making the right decision. I had always been someone who goes all in—I would overthink, overplan, and overanalyze. I had the chance to go for a run, but I decided to take a rest day instead of modifying my plans with a walk. I knew that walking with heel pain would worsen the situation, and it wasn't worth the risk of being sidelined with two upcoming races and training I had come to appreciate.

Over the years, I've made many mistakes by failing to think ahead. I hadn't considered the "what ifs," and there were too many times I wished I could have had a do-over. It's easy to look back and pinpoint what might have caused my pain. In the moment, I felt the pain and made the smart decision to stop before things got worse. Foreseeing issues and changing course ahead of time is challenging, but I've learned to pause—rather than regret a decision I wish I hadn't made.

So, I worked on my mindset, shifting from *"Can I really do this?"* to *"Let's get out there and give it a whirl."* I joined Strava challenges for the 5K and 10K, as well as a 30-hour activity challenge. When I ran five and a half miles outside while staying with my in-laws, I played faster-paced music and ran up and down the streets until I reached my goal. I didn't focus on the time or pace; I checked the time occasionally just to see how far I had gone, but I truly didn't care about my pace. That run really turned things around for me mentally. I felt such a high in the hours after finishing. I had run that distance many times before, but this run felt significant!

I started to get excited about my runs, appreciating the beautiful landscaping and gorgeous homes as I ran through the golf community. When I went out for my six-mile run a week later, I did the same thing—admiring the perfect blue sky and the beauty around me. I felt determined to complete those six miles and experienced the same rush of excitement from pushing myself. When I stopped the watch at six miles, I saw I had finished in just under an hour—faster and farther than I had gone in a long time!

Everything was coming together.

On February 20, I ran the Freezing 4 Miler with Jeff. I had signed up for this race on a whim, without really considering how *"freezing"* it would be. I just wanted to race and get back to trail running after a long break. I didn't care how long it took me to run the four miles—it was all about the experience. I layered up and met Jeff at the Rocky River Mastick picnic area, where the race was held. I kept telling Jeff to run his own race and meet me at the finish line, but he insisted on staying with me.

Shortly before the start, I removed my neck gaiter because it was interfering with my breathing, and I felt comfortable in my layers despite the 25-degree temperature at the start. I didn't know our pace as we ran together, but the mile markers were helpful.

Passing mile 1, I realized we had another mile before turning back to the finish line. Jeff was very encouraging, telling me we were pacing well and that my breathing sounded good. With 75 participants, we finished in 43:07—somewhere in the middle. I was just happy to be out there racing again.

The next day, I made some mistakes.

I had previously talked about how you can sometimes see a decision looming and have a moment to change course for the better. But other times, there's no space to pause or consider your options. When you take the wrong turn, hindsight hits you like a smack to the forehead—for something so easily avoidable.

I went to the JCC the day after the 4 Miler since I had woken up early and would be watching my grandchildren later. I had a mile repeat run on my training plan (which didn't account for the 4-mile race), and after doing my stretching routine, I got on the treadmill. Within two minutes, I felt that familiar Achilles pain. I knew continuing would be a bad move. I switched to the elliptical and maintained a moderate pace for 12 minutes, but the pain persisted. I then moved to the recumbent bike, which felt fine.

I texted Jeff later about my attempt at running, and we discussed where the pain was located. I could almost hear the steam coming out of him as he texted that I should have taken the day off—**PERIOD.** He emphasized that I shouldn't have expected to do any speed work or running the day after a race in extreme cold. I also shouldn't have worked out first thing in the morning without allowing myself recovery time.

Reflecting on my actions, I wished I'd had the wisdom to stay in bed that morning and skip the gym. I promised myself I would take a full day off after any race—regardless of the distance or how easy it seemed. From now on, I would use hindsight to avoid past mistakes and make better decisions.

About two weeks before the Jerusalem 10K, I started training for the Towpath Half. It was great to see so many weeks checked off my training plan, but I knew I still had a lot of work to do. I felt ready for the 10K—both physically and mentally. During a seven-mile treadmill run, I felt like I could've gone a little longer—a rare feeling. The training plan called for 9–11 mile long runs, and our virtual training sessions focused on mobility and strength work—no tapering, as I typically would do before a race.

During a 10-mile long run on the treadmill, I pictured myself standing with Kimi at the Towpath Half starting line, excited to race together. I also imagined clear skies and 55 degrees! We had talked about how much fun we would have, taking selfies with my two sons visiting Cleveland, who had decided to run the half as well. The excitement in the air promised a new experience—as no two half marathons are ever the same. Imagining those pre-race moments helped motivate me through the 10-mile run. I wanted to do the run anyway, but I hadn't been feeling *it* until I visualized that starting line setting.

The day before the 10K, I felt race-ready! I knew I had trained for this race for 23 weeks, and I was excited. The forecast predicted light rain throughout the week, but I knew there was nothing I could do about it. Whatever the weather would be, I accepted it. It would be cold, but I would have the warm fuzzies from being at this event—where I would undoubtedly see many people I hadn't seen in ages—running through the city of Jerusalem with my youngest daughter as my running mate.

I would enjoy this 10K as an *experience* rather than the race I had originally planned. I had been under the weather for the past 10 days, and considering the wet pavement and predicted rain, I decided not to focus on achieving a PR. I would give it my all, but I'd be smart and mindful of the ground conditions to avoid slipping or getting too winded. I would face the four hills and tackle them based on how I felt physically and the surface conditions—without the panic I felt during previous Jerusalem 10Ks.

The time wouldn't matter, and I wouldn't look at my watch to check my pace. This was about using everything I had worked for over the past 23 weeks and crossing the finish line with a smile—knowing all my hard work had paid off.

More than five months of mile repeats, speed intervals, long runs, and easy runs culminated in a wet, cold, and challenging race. I had trained hard and mentally prepared for the hills, but on that day, I just didn't have it in me. It had rained steadily from the night before through 7:30 on race morning, with the 10K scheduled for

9:45. Fortunately, the sun emerged, transforming the dreary gray skies into picturesque clouds and blue.

We left before 6:00 and drove to the racecourse in two cars—Gary took Liat, our friends Michele and Bella, while my son drove with his older siblings. Gary dropped us off to dry out in a nearby mall while he parked and stayed closer to the course for his 7:30 5K start. The rain returned just as we enjoyed an early breakfast at a café a few minutes from the starting line. (Earlier that week, I had reserved a 90-minute slot at the café between Gary's 5K start and our 10K.) Gary arrived soaking wet, followed shortly by Yonatan, who had completed his half marathon.

I panicked... Should I wear the rain jacket I brought, or would I be overdressed? I chose the extra layer, which proved wise—it was 40 degrees outside, but felt more like 30 with the rain. The weather prevented the usual mingling of crowds at the starting line, where we often bump into familiar faces. Before we knew it, it was 9:15, and Liat and I headed to the starting line, waiting for the official start.

Off we went, doing our best to move with the crowd and find our position within the first two kilometers. I felt the effects of the cold I had been fighting for the past week and a half, and my lungs were struggling. As we approached the bottom of Betzalel Street, where the first significant hill began, it felt as if the hill were daring me to run up it. I channeled my trail runner self and started trotting up, but halfway, I switched to a walk. I just couldn't do it. I didn't have the energy to run the rest of that hill, so I walked.

I felt guilty for not being able to run up that hill (and the three subsequent hills along the course) after training for them for so long. Still, I knew I was doing my best under the circumstances—cold, rain, and not feeling well. I ran as much as I could on Jaffa Street and other flat areas, but I walked every hill, feeling defeated.

I had set two goals for the race and didn't come close to either. I hadn't run the entire course, hills included, and I hadn't achieved a personal record. I glanced at my watch occasionally to check our time, but eventually shrugged it off, realizing this race wasn't about personal records or finishing faster than my previous 10Ks. In the end, we finished the 10K in 1:11:20—not bad considering I walked the hills.

Liat was an amazing running partner, sticking with me even when I told her more than once to leave me and run her own race. She insisted we were doing this race together, and that mindset made me realize what this race was truly about. I had started my fitness journey for various reasons—to lose weight, get stronger and leaner—but more importantly, to be the best wife, mother, and grandmother I could be.

Liat had taken up running less than two years before and had become a superstar in her own right. She understood that I valued my health and made it a priority, so running a destination 10K alongside her was the highlight of an otherwise low morning. We were fortunate that the rain stopped before we started the 10K, and it really only drizzled until we were two kilometers from the finish. Then it poured again.

We lingered around the muddy fields of Sacher Park, waiting for Seth to finish his marathon. As miserable as I felt, I knew I couldn't leave before seeing him complete his race. It was Friday morning, and I had a house full of guests to cook for—but we had come to this race together, and we would leave together. Gary, our kids, and I stood by the sidelines, waiting for him and his friend to approach the finish line. When we saw them coming, we cheered at the top of our lungs!

I had two days to rest before returning to training for the half marathon. I completed a nine-mile long run and felt fine, then took the next day as a rest day since we were flying back to Cleveland. My cold seemed to improve, and I felt stronger than I had during the 10K, but I began to feel anxious and nervous about the race. *Could I really do this half?!*

Deep down, I knew I could. I had already completed nine-, ten-, and eleven-mile long runs, plus three previous half marathons. I imagined myself at the starting line with Kimi, picturing the feeling of accomplishment and the glory that comes with crossing a finish line. I visualized the mile 1, mile 2, and mile 12 markers—each one drawing me closer to the end. I had to stop thinking about what would happen *if* I couldn't go further and start thinking about how I would feel *when* I did.

This half wasn't about time or pace. My previous half marathons had been about that, and I would always be proud of those results. The first half wasn't about time since I had nothing to compare it to—it was about achieving something beyond my expectations (and I had a great time doing it). The second half had been more focused on time, and things were going well until the heat got to me, causing me to go down for a bit before getting back up to finish. Had I not lost those 17 minutes, I would have achieved a personal record—but I couldn't dwell on what could have been when I was satisfied with how the race went overall.

The third half was meant to be about time—and it ended up being a PR by 10 seconds—but it was a harder race that required more challenging training. At the time, I hadn't thought I would—or could—do another half, because I didn't feel ready to invest the effort required for long runs. Yet here I was, having managed to complete them.

I had an 11-mile long run scheduled for the last Sunday before the half, and I decided to approach it with excitement and determination. I was going to make this run the one that set me up for the race. On race day, I would be ready to put one foot in front of the other and remember all the long runs I had done—knowing I could complete the race.

However, that Sunday, as I prepared for the 11-mile long run, I woke up with a deep, horrible cough that made me suspect bronchitis or even pneumonia. I had felt fine the week before and was sure I had finally recovered from the upper respiratory issue I'd had while in Israel. I had been sleeping well most nights that week, even with the jet lag, and felt physically and mentally ready for the half. If anything, I was more nervous about the 11-mile long run than the race itself.

But the cough felt serious—and it sounded concerning. My husband suggested I take a COVID test, and within seconds, I received a positive result. A PCR test later confirmed it, and I felt terrible. I didn't know what was worse—being sick or having to tell Kimi I couldn't do the half the following week.

I called her to explain I had COVID, and we agreed not to panic or assume the worst, as I was confident I would feel better within a few days. She was understanding, even offering to turn it into a half marathon walk if we couldn't manage a mix of running and walking. I used the next several days to rest and hoped to be well enough for race day, but by Thursday, I realized I wouldn't be in any shape to race. I got winded just walking up the stairs and often had to lie down to rest.

I could still do virtual training sessions with Jeff, focusing on stretching and gentle yoga moves, but no treadmill walks or intense workouts. I felt terrible telling Kimi I wouldn't be able to do the half with her. I had hoped and prayed that I would recover within a week—but it just wasn't going to happen.

She assured me we would have other halves to run together, and I promised to hold her to that. I knew she would do great at the Towpath Half, having watched her train hard for it—but it was still disappointing to know I'd be at home on race day.

On the morning of my first DNS (Did Not Start), I left the house for the first time in a week and went for a walk. I walked from my house down the street to the end—a third of a mile—and I felt awful. It took me 20 minutes to walk that distance, and another 20 minutes to walk back. I felt discouraged by how long it took. I knew that healing takes time and can't be rushed, yet I still felt like a failure.

As I walked (or strolled) for those 40 minutes, I reflected on what it meant to DNS. I had heard the term before, but it had never applied to me. I had always completed my races—even the Cleveland Half Marathon, where I was on the ground for 17 minutes before managing to get up and walk slowly to the finish line. I'd had a few DNSs due to weather cancellations, but this was the first time I was the reason—and that really sucked.

My friend, a cardiologist, warned me that stepping onto the starting line at the Towpath would be a terrible decision, and deep down, I knew I had to listen. The choice to DNS was made with a clear but aching head, and even though I had made the decision before race day, it was still hard. Throughout the week, I had hoped I could lower my pace, mix in walking, or even walk the entire course. But I knew, deep down, that would be a mistake I'd regret long after the race. I didn't want to stop mid-race and be stuck—unable to go any further or, worse, collapse.

I knew running would still be there. Whether it took a week or a month to get back to it, I would run again. And when I did, I would appreciate my comeback even more.

That comeback went smoothly. I took another walk outside and really listened to my body. I knew better than to focus on my pace or compete with myself. Feeling fully recovered, I did my first run on the treadmill while we were in Orlando, Florida for Passover—and I took it nice and slow. I decided to try the MAF heart rate training method, since it's known for building sustainable pace, but I wanted to approach my return to running with caution and common sense.

I tried it for three days and gave up—perhaps too hastily—as I found it incredibly difficult to keep my heart rate under 132 during my runs. My average pace improved slightly, but running at that rate felt more like crawling. I had read up on the MAF method and believed it to be a great way to enhance athletic performance, but it just didn't seem right for me.

In May, I found myself on a roller coaster of lost-and-found motivation. Earlier that month, I enjoyed the freedom of not following a training plan again. I was running four times a week, with longer runs scheduled on Wednesdays and 2–3 miles on other days. I liked being in control—choosing the type of run and the pace. It felt like I was "back," running for quality rather than quantity. I was getting more out of my runs, which might not have seemed far in distance but were higher in intensity. I even considered running the River Run Half Marathon in September with a friend… shocking, right?!

My workouts with Jeff increased in intensity, and I started using heavier weights, making me feel stronger and more empowered. But by the end of May, I hit a wall. One morning, I just didn't want to run. I didn't know what was wrong, but I felt off for the first hour after waking up. I had planned to drive to Brecksville for a few miles, figuring a destination run would be worth the drive. I laid out my clothes the night before to avoid last-minute outfit decisions.

I reluctantly put on a long-sleeve dry-fit shirt and capris, not realizing it was already nearing 68 degrees outside by the time I headed out. I drove with mixed feelings about whether the longer top was a good idea, but I refused to turn around to change. I wasn't feeling upbeat as I started the run. I held back my pace, but after the first mile, I began to get into it.

With my earphones not working and no music to listen to, I made a point to absorb everything the run had to offer. I waved and mouthed hello to fellow walkers and runners and took in the greenery around me—the trees, leaves, and grass. I felt my *mojo* returning in the second half of mile 2 and picked up the pace. I reached the bridge parking lot and continued on the towpath until I hit three miles and pressed the stop button. It was enough.

The run transformed from "yuck" to "yeah," and I felt good for not giving in to my morning reluctance—and for not turning back when I realized I was unprepared, both in clothing and music. What started as a C run quickly turned into a B+.

The next morning, I woke up wanting to work out. I wanted to take a walk—either before my training session with Jeff or sometime mid-morning after. The weather app predicted rain for the next two hours, so I stayed in bed and relaxed. I ended up walking two miles on the treadmill in my basement before the training session, and even though I could have done more, I kept it short to avoid overdoing it.

I continued focusing on the intensity of my runs and workouts rather than just effort. Jeff's workouts had me doing upper body strength exercises, some leg work using the bench I bought for my basement gym, and TRX with aerobic movements mixed in to elevate my heart rate. I realized my running intensity had been lacking. Granted, my speed interval runs were becoming more intense as I pushed through higher-paced bursts, but I needed to focus on intensity during my road runs as well.

One Wednesday in Rocky River, while running with Jeff, I paid closer attention to my intensity. I let him record our run on his watch, so I had no idea how far or fast we were going. It felt great to be outside and push myself! I monitored my breathing, making sure I wasn't huffing and puffing, and I focused on picking up my feet to avoid dragging along the trails.

In June, I diagnosed myself with *multiple running personality disorder.* One minute, I'd be ready to run—dressed, double-laced, and blasting fast-paced music. Then I'd start the run with mixed feelings, but after a quarter mile, I'd be fully engaged—physically and mentally. There were also times I knew I had to run but felt dread or a sense of obligation rather than excitement. I'd complete the run, sometimes forgetting my initial reluctance and feeling glad I did it. Other times, the run didn't go well, and I'd beat myself up about it—for a few minutes, or longer.

It's all mental. I knew my mind needed to sync with my body for a good run from start to finish. Running is never exact. I could run three miles four days a week, but no two—or three, or four—runs are ever the same. My heart rate would vary. My pace would change. My gait and stride would differ.

And that variation is great—because if I ran the same distance, pace, and time every single run, it would get boring fast. I never wanted to get bored with running. I might experience occasional dips in motivation, but I knew running gave me something no other exercise could: an adrenaline rush and a sense of accomplishment.

In the past, I had run to train for races, challenge myself to a personal best, raise money for charity, or lose weight. I've been running for seven years, and I've evolved as a runner during that time. With this disorder now officially self-diagnosed, I knew I had to run just for the joy of running. I wouldn't focus on a specific time or pace. I needed to *just run*—upcoming races included—without checking my watch every few minutes, and be okay with the outcome.

I did something significant on June 13: I canceled my membership with Weight Watchers—now called WW.

Much of my journey had focused more on fitness and less on weight maintenance turned weight loss efforts. It was easier to blog about training for a race or my workouts with Jeff than to confront the struggles I've had with the scale since I was 17. I struggled with my weight and poor self-esteem due to the extra pounds. I tried countless diets and quick fixes in my late teens and 20s, and my GI system paid the price. I watched the scale fluctuate like a bad week on the stock market—losing 10 pounds and regaining 15. It was, indeed, a battle of the bulge for over two decades.

I finally got serious in 2006 while planning my oldest daughter's Bat Mitzvah. I wanted to look good in a specific dress and knew I needed to lose 10–15 pounds to pull it off. I joined Weight Watchers (somewhat of an annual event!) and managed to lose a substantial amount of weight that I kept off for several years. I started working out to maintain my weight, and that story was told in the beginning of this book. I shifted my focus on WW from a diet to a lifestyle, and it worked—for a long time.

I achieved Lifetime status in 2011 and earned the gold key that had eluded me during many previous attempts that never lasted more than a week or two. I continued to track diligently as I started working out with Jeff, who not only changed my life through running and training, but also helped me with my nutrition. Together, we realized I couldn't eat the same way every day. I resisted trying certain foods for too long—like red meat and healthy oils—fearing they would contradict WW's ideals.

As my body changed over the years with added muscle, I panicked when the scale went up, berating myself for allowing it and letting the WW program determine my success. I changed my target weight several times to give myself grace and avoid the shame of being "over" the number and having to pay a fee as punishment. When I decided to cancel my membership, I knew I weighed more than I did at my daughter's Bat Mitzvah and was above my original target weight.

For too long, I felt shame and disappointment because I let something external dictate my success, believing I was a failure for not meeting its requirements. I often skipped weigh-ins when I saw an unfavorable number. It became the diet I had promised myself not to view as such, and it stopped feeling like a lifestyle.

When I achieved Lifetime status in 2011, I vowed never to cancel my subscription—convinced I would become a statistic and regain the weight on my own. But ultimately, I decided to cancel my WW membership and go my own way.

The truth is, I wasn't alone. I was following an eating plan that worked for me. While I might not have seen results on the scale, I knew it was the right approach. I recognized that the scale didn't determine my success—but it had dictated it for too long, affecting my self-esteem.

As I canceled my membership, I felt a weight lift off me—ironically. Before I clicked "yes," I was offered a free month to "stick it out." But I had been sticking it out far longer than I should have. I still believe the program works for those who commit to it—and I had committed for a long time. But now, I had faith in what I was doing with Jeff regarding nutrition and fitness. And if I ever wanted to return, it would still be there.

On June 3, I ran the Full Moon 2-Miler—and I had the pictures to prove it. My time was 18:19:45! There were three photos: two of Jeff and me running together, and a third of me sprinting toward the finish line alongside another female runner.

At first, I cringed when I saw them in my email from Hermes. But after a second look, I noticed how I was moving my arms like the Bionic Woman. I hesitated to post the pictures on Facebook or Instagram because I thought I looked terrible. Initially, I saw my knee-length shorts and pink tank top, focusing on how large my hips looked. I thought I should have worn a looser top and capris to draw less attention to my thighs and knees.

However, upon further examination, I realized I was running toward the finish line—arms in motion, legs powering forward. My upper arms looked somewhat muscular (thanks, Jeff, for those amazing workouts), and despite being exposed, my knees actually looked defined. A third look revealed my determination and focus—and I noticed I was ahead of the woman next to me, who appeared to be in "better" shape.

Looking at those pictures, I recognized how easy it is to focus on the negative and criticize oneself. But by taking another look, I could see the positive and appreciate that moment as something beautiful.

Ironically, I found a picture of myself from the Full Moon race in August 2021—wearing a similar outfit and sporting that same focused expression near the finish line. In that photo, I saw an athlete. And that's not a word I use lightly. I was in the moment, running with determination and purpose. I was a 53-year-old wife, mother, and grandmother doing something I truly enjoyed—stronger physically, mentally, and emotionally. That photo captured me thriving in the moment. I wasn't thinking about how I looked (I didn't even know the picture was taken!). I was running alongside hundreds of others who couldn't care less about my knees in those shorts or what the scale said that morning.

By the end of June, my intensity level seemed to return. My runs were going well, and while I wasn't focused on pace or time, I was excited about my progress. I felt back in action, and my mental toughness had returned. Granted, I was now seven years older than when I first started running, and my body had changed. I was not the same runner I was seven years ago. But the drive I had rediscovered—that spark—was the same as when I first took up running. And I wanted to hold onto it as long as possible.

I had been using a running journal since October 2020, filled with notes and stats from each run, and it was time for a new book. As a writer, I appreciated how the journal allowed me to record and reflect. I included distance, overall pace, weather (if the run was outside), and a few lines about the run.

Reviewing that first journal, I noticed many entries focused more on how I felt physically or how I wasn't fully engaged in the run. It seemed more like a rant than a true reflection. During some treadmill runs, I recorded how I hadn't felt great but still reported my pace. I didn't realize at the time that I was making excuses rather than sharing insights about my runs. Re-reading the journal allowed me to revisit those runs through the details. Unfortunately, most memories weren't as positive as I would have liked. I wondered if I had written more about what those runs meant to me—rather than complaining about foot pain or poor sleep—I might have reflected with a better perspective.

In the last month or so, I noticed a shift in my mindset regarding my intensity level, and I began writing more about the routes I took and how I felt after completing them. My running journal evolved from posts reflecting a weakened mindset to a true journal. I started recording runs with stats *and* notes about their significance, enabling me to look back and recall them with an *"oh yeah... I remember that"* feeling. I was excited to start a new journal. I couldn't wait to share my runs—whether for my eyes only or to share with others. I knew that journaling about my runs could encompass so much more than the runs themselves, allowing me to genuinely express my physical and mental feelings as I began each run—without turning them into excuses or confessions.

In early July, I recognized that I was facing another setback with my running. I realized it was 99% mental. Yes, there had been a long period of canceled races and gym closures due to the pandemic, but something had convinced me I was slower and weaker than in my earlier running years. Furthermore, I had lost the joy I once felt every time I ran. I was holding myself back, both physically and mentally, telling myself I wasn't capable of running further or faster. I had been going through the motions of running—feeling like it was something I *had* to do, rather than something I enjoyed.

It took time, many runs, and deep conversations with Jeff, who assured me I *would* rediscover the joy of running—but that it was something I had to seek out. Earlier in the year, I had decided to let go of the numbers and run for the sheer joy of it. This shift helped me focus on being out there, doing it simply because I could.

My internal struggle with the scale hadn't helped my running, especially since I was convinced the extra weight was hindering my performance. But once I decided to quit WW and stop being a slave to the scale, I felt a sense of freedom—and within a week, that freedom positively impacted my approach to running.

I began looking forward to my runs instead of dreading them. I warmed up properly, eager to do the various stretches, knowing they would prepare my body. I chose to run outside instead of on the treadmill because outdoor running offered an awareness I wouldn't have gained indoors. I started to take in my surroundings—the people walking their dogs, riding bikes, the sounds of car horns and barking dogs. After each run, I felt a joy I had been missing for far too long.

I wasn't trying to go back to the runner I was in 2015. I refused to let my stats on Runkeeper dictate my success or failure. Letting go of the numbers allowed me to appreciate running for what it gave me—the feeling of conquering a big hill by jogging up it, refusing to let my lack of confidence convince me I could only walk.

As I began training for the River Run Half, I faced a challenging summer on the medical front. Earlier in the year, I was diagnosed with focal/microscopic colitis, a chronic inflammatory bowel disease affecting the large bowel. I was prescribed medication to manage it, and I've learned to live with it—thankfully, it's not a severe case.

In April, I consulted a rheumatologist about some autoimmune concerns. I had been diagnosed with vitiligo in my early 20s, but the cause remained unclear. Along with Raynaud's phenomenon in my feet and a positive test for an undetermined blood disorder, I was referred to a wonderful doctor at the Cleveland Clinic. She tested me for various rheumatic and blood disorders. Thankfully, she ruled out lupus and most serious conditions, but I did test positive for a concerning clotting disorder, which prompted a referral to a vascular doctor.

During that appointment, I mentioned that three years prior, I underwent testing for Fibromuscular Dysplasia (FMD), but it wasn't clear if I had it—and I was due for repeat testing in 2024. (I had experienced abdominal pain that led me to my internist, who ordered an ultrasound noting an ectatic aorta and possible FMD in my carotid and iliac arteries.) While the vascular doctor didn't find the clotting disorder alarming, he ordered ultrasounds to check the areas previously scanned in 2019.

An abdominal ultrasound revealed that my aorta's ectasia had progressed, leading to a referral to a colleague specializing in FMD. After reviewing the results of my head-to-pelvis CTA and ultrasound imaging, I received an official diagnosis: Fibromuscular Dysplasia. FMD is a somewhat rare vascular disease that narrows medium-sized arteries in the circulatory system, leading to stenosis, aneurysm, and dissection. I had it in my carotid, iliac, and renal arteries, with some questionable narrowing in neighboring arteries I hadn't even known existed—hepatic, splenic, celiac.

My doctor has been an amazing source of support, providing reading materials about FMD and a few restrictions: no lifting over 30 pounds, no roller coasters, and avoiding sudden neck or head movements—to reduce the risk of potential artery events. When I told her I run a few times a week and had a half marathon coming up, she said I could continue running as long as I felt okay, but I needed to monitor my heart rate and avoid pushing my pace too much. She also instructed me to take 81 mg of baby aspirin daily (for both my clotting disorder and FMD) and get annual ultrasounds to track any changes.

The diagnosis was frightening, especially the restrictions on weight lifting and the caution needed during my runs. I had just ordered a pair of 30-pound dumbbells the week before my appointment with Dr. McCarthy—only to find that the 30-pound limit meant total weight, not per dumbbell! I tried not to let FMD control my life, but it lingered in the back of my mind—warning me that a plank or push-up might be too much, or that pushing my pace could be risky.

Still, I continued training for the River Run, excited to run it with my friend Frankie. I had done the race twice before and enjoyed the course. This time, I approached my training with enthusiasm, following the plan with positivity. The plan included a long run each week, increasing by half a mile weekly. I did as much running outside as possible and felt my intensity improve—or so I thought. My paces were in the 10–11 minute-per-mile range, but I could feel the increase in effort. I used faster-paced music to stay motivated and stuck to planned routes for each outdoor run, which helped keep my mindset strong.

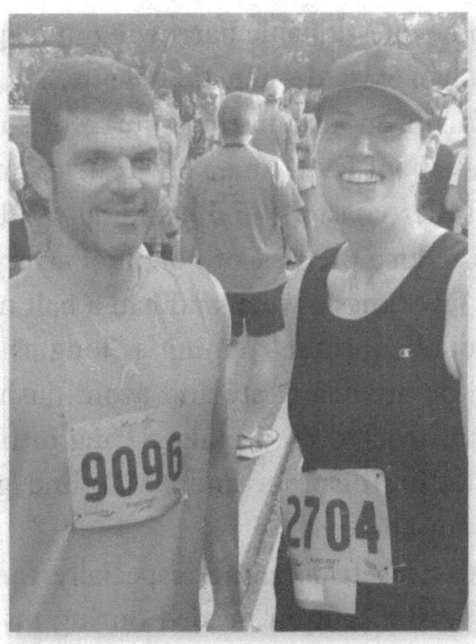

© 2016 Gary Weiss

In late July, Jeff and I ran Adam's Run in Peninsula. Afterward, I mentioned to him that I felt out of shape. I had struggled to keep up with him during the first mile on the challenging trails. Although we weren't running super fast, the intensity made it hard for me to control my breathing. It felt like the run took forever; we'd only gone three-quarters of a mile, but I was convinced we'd already passed the first mile. Was I really that out of shape?

And yet, I enjoyed the run—I really did. I even liked getting my feet wet as we ran along the streams. I trotted up the hills and reached the top, continuing with my run. At one point, Jeff told me to take the lead, and I found my way along the trails with him just a few feet behind. I felt less out of shape as I led us, thinking maybe I was just out of *practice* rather than out of *shape*. I hadn't done more than a handful of trail runs with Jeff that spring or summer due to increased travel, and he had warned me that this particular run would be more challenging.

One day at the supermarket, I bumped into an acquaintance from my old Weight Watchers meetings. I shared that I had quit WW a few months earlier and hadn't heard from our meeting leader or the WW national office. She recalled how I used to be a regular treadmill walker and asked if I still did that. I told her I had taken up running in 2015 and was still doing it—along with twice-a-week training sessions.

She complimented how great I looked and noted that I had maintained my weight since we last saw each other. I thanked her and returned the compliment—she had always seemed trim and put together. Later that day, I reflected on her comment. Realizing I hadn't seen her since 2012, I momentarily slipped into the mindset of *"I weigh so much more than I did when you last saw me."* For a moment—and it *was* just a moment—I let the scale define my worth. But I quickly redirected my thoughts toward something more positive.

I reminded myself: from her perspective, I looked good. I was wearing a fitted top and cute skirt—the same type of outfit I wore when we were WW meeting buddies. She didn't know that I hadn't worn that outfit in months and had only decided that morning that I finally felt okay putting it on.

I had a nine-mile long run on my half marathon training plan that, despite my preparation, didn't go as planned. I had my clothes and shoes ready, stretched, reviewed my route, and even read a note about handling tough moments. Music was playing in my earphones, and I felt ready. I followed the route precisely, but as I neared eight miles, I felt my legs starting to give out.

I had been practicing *managing myself*—something Jeff suggested I memorize—meaning staying aware of my body while keeping focus. It meant slowing down if I felt I was going too fast. But despite that awareness, I realized my run had turned into a jog. My lips felt numb, and the wobbly sensation in my legs wouldn't go away. I pressed the stop button at the eight-mile mark and mentally kicked myself. I had wanted to complete the full nine miles. I was prepared—physically and mentally—but my body said no.

It didn't like being pushed that hard. So I turned to Jeff for support. When I told him about the numb lips and the unsteady legs, he suggested we change the plan. Some train for half marathons with one long run a week. I had trained that way for my first half, and it had worked well—but that was six years ago. Jeff recommended we switch to back-to-back days of running for the rest of my training. I was willing to do whatever it took to get there. I wasn't aiming for a PR with this half, nor focused on a specific time. I just wanted to do my best—and if the training plan needed to change, I was okay with that.

Two weeks before the race, I spent a good part of a Sunday morning soul-searching. I never thought I'd do another half marathon, but I had signed up with the hope of running it with Frankie. Unfortunately, she came down with a nasty flu and lost too much training time to commit—even after she started feeling better. Knowing I would now run this half alone, part of me wanted to cancel. But deep down, I felt ready. I had worked hard on my mindset, and I was determined to do this race no matter what.

That mindset shift was significant. Earlier in the year, I had struggled with motivation. But something clicked—and I felt like I'd fallen in love with running again, or at least *most* of the time. I learned to psyche myself up mentally before long runs and no longer felt that freaked-out feeling when running outside. During my post-run walks, I reminded myself that I *got* to do that run—that it was a privilege, not a burden. There were times I felt too tired or overwhelmed mid-run, but instead of stopping my watch, I channeled Jeff's advice: manage myself. That meant slowing down or giving myself verbal encouragement that I could finish.

I had two more weeks to prepare—physically and mentally—for this half marathon, for this experience. I had done the work. I was conditioned to show up at the starting line and do my thing.

Even though I thought I was okay with running the half on my own, I still wanted a racing buddy. I found one in Tracy, a member of the Facebook MRTT/SRTT running page, and we made plans to meet at the race and run together as much as we could. I had my race bib mailed to me, so I was all set.

Or was I?

The week before the half, I became frustrated after a "bad" run. I was supposed to run five and a half miles, but it didn't go as expected. I had stretched and was mentally prepared to follow the route I'd designed on Runkeeper. I left the house ready to complete the run. I planned to run five and a half miles that day and another five the next, splitting a ten-and-a-half-mile long run.

I felt fine as I started out on my neighborhood streets, telling myself I could finish before the predicted rain...

About three miles in, I felt my right leg give out. It was a gradual issue—it started in the back of my right leg and moved down through my knee to my right calf. I kept telling myself to manage it because I still had two miles left. I slowed my pace as I headed onto one of my neighborhood streets that stretches a full mile, and that's when my right leg locked up at 3.34 miles. I pressed the stop button on my Strava and, with tears in my eyes, walked/limped the three blocks home.

I was in serious pain, questioning if I had jeopardized my race. I texted Jeff to tell him about the aborted run and waited for his advice. Would he tell me to push through? Would he say I could take a break and taper until the race?

He didn't say either of those things.

He told me to "find her."

I didn't understand what he meant.

He reminded me of the woman who had crawled up a muddy incline and made it to the top at her first Spartan race. Jeff assured me I was physically ready for the half—but I needed to work on the mental aspect. If I didn't feel like doing the race (I did!), then I shouldn't do it.

It felt like we were playing Truth or Dare, and he was daring me to race while I had to face the truth: Did I still want to do this race?

Definitely.

I didn't care about my pace; I just wanted to participate. I had worked hard for this race and wouldn't let fear or doubt take over. I searched for 'her' and tried to find her.

I thought about the wife and mother of five who, eight years ago, decided to do something for herself. I remembered the self-proclaimed klutz who jumped over a fire pit and crawled under barbed wire—not once, but twice. I considered the couch potato who bravely shared her wish to run and ended up with a drawer full of race medals and bibs, along with tales of 5Ks, 10Ks, half marathons, Spartan races, and trail races.

That 'her' was me.

And I needed to channel her when things got tough on race day.

A blackened toe. Chafing from a fanny pack. Rain. Tired calves and quads at mile 3. Humidity. Two hours of sleep. GI issues. Receiving my medal at the finish line. The picture with Tracy post-race, where we smiled ear to ear. Running toward the finish line without a care about the clock.

It would be easy to focus on the negatives of my third River Run half marathon, but it truly was a mixed bag. I couldn't allow myself to dwell on criticisms about an experience that left me feeling so high.

I drove to Berea with plenty of time to make multiple trips to the bathroom and stretch. The rain poured as I drove, and I knew it wouldn't let up. I really didn't want to run in the rain—I hated getting wet and then driving home in drenched clothes—but I had no choice. I wasn't going to turn around and skip the race. Tracy was counting on me, and more importantly, I was counting on me.

Rain or no rain, there was no backing out.

I had trained hard for this race, and the past two weeks had been especially challenging. I pushed everything aside as I drove in the rain, giving myself grace to run with the sole intention of finishing.

I met up with Tracy in the parking lot and got to know her better before the race. I debated whether to wear my rain jacket. Several runners had ponchos, others wore their dri-fit best. I decided to tie my jacket around my waist in case I needed it for extra protection.

The gun went off, and Tracy and I started the race. We ran the first few miles together, sticking to our plan of a 10:30–11-minute-mile pace. We were doing great—until I felt that familiar soreness in my calf. We switched to short walking intervals for another mile or so, and then I told Tracy to go ahead and run her own race. I didn't want to hold her back and sensed we might fall behind our time goal of 2:25.

I ran as much as I could and walked as briefly as possible. It was lonely running without anyone to encourage me, but I managed to get through it, mile by mile. I crossed the finish line in 2:37:39 and suddenly didn't feel bad about my time—or how I finished.

Another DNS (Did Not Start)… my second ever, and within six

months! When I signed up for the Full Moon 5 Miler at North Chagrin, I marked it on my calendar with mixed excitement and trepidation. A five-mile trail race was something I had never done, and I'd been told it was a challenging course with significant elevation and steep hills. I figured I'd participate since I would be in Cleveland in September and wanted to race as much as possible.

A week before the race, I realized it was scheduled just two days after my River Run half! I knew it would be a mistake to do a trail race right after a half, regardless of how much walking I had mixed in or how long it took me to finish. I had to take a week off after the half to recover, so even the idea of walking the 5 Miler was too much. My right calf had been sore since the race, and I had been doing all kinds of rehab: stretching, Icy Cold patches, foam rolling, the massage gun, infrared light, and plain rest.

On the morning of the trail race, I struggled to walk around the house and knew that attempting five miles on a trail would hinder my recovery. I couldn't believe I had messed up. My intentions were good when I signed up for the Full Moon months before deciding to do the half. I had genuinely planned to do that trail race and had no reason not to… until I decided to go ahead with a fourth half marathon that summer. I knew deep down that staying home on that Tuesday evening was the right decision, but it didn't feel good. I wanted to race, and had I not been in the middle of recovery, I could have done it. The hills might have been a challenge, but I could have managed them—and it would have been great to run a course of trails I had never experienced.

I knew there would be other races in my future, and I was confident that running would be waiting for me once I fully recovered.

As I celebrated turning 54 on September 30, I recognized I wasn't the same person I had been when I first took up running. I used to focus on pace and was often my own worst enemy. I didn't consider what other female runners my age were doing; I made it a contest against myself, comparing my performances from one race to another. I didn't realize how much pressure I was putting on myself until the pandemic reduced the number of races.

At 54, I lacked the innocence I had at 46, but I had gained

newfound awareness, and my outlook shifted from focusing on pace or time. I signed up for races because I wanted to, not for the thrill of seeing my name in the top three. Sure, that would have been amazing—and it was incredible the few times I placed in the top three—but it wasn't about the prize. It has always been about the accomplishment of doing something I never imagined I could do and how I felt when I finished.

My 54-year-old self wanted to run simply because I could—not for a medal, a specific distance, or a time. I wasn't racing against myself. All I had to do was start my run and finish it; the part in the middle was up to me. I could choose my route and run at whatever pace I wanted; it wasn't a competition.

Back in Israel, I was walking with my younger daughter in downtown Jerusalem when she told me how glad she was that I was dedicated to working out. I agreed but expressed my wish that I had started earlier. I noticed my parents struggling with their walkers a few feet behind us and told her it was never too late to start.

Later that day, I reflected on our conversation and asked myself why I was doing all of this. I had begun my fitness journey later in life, but I was proof that it was never too late. I wanted to be active at 64 and 74. I had adopted a more active lifestyle primarily to feel good and stay healthy, but I quickly realized I genuinely enjoyed it. I was also motivated by the alternative—I didn't want to struggle with health issues or move slower if I could prevent that.

I decided to participate in the Miami Half Marathon in January 2023 with my younger brother. He had walked the race many times with his wife, but I had never been able to join them because I was either in Cleveland or Israel. When he shared the date, I saw that Gary and I would be in Florida visiting our parents and close friends, so I promptly signed up. We weren't sure if we would walk the course or do a run/walk, since my brother wasn't much of a runner... yet.

I also planned to run the Jerusalem Half Marathon that following March because I wanted to try something different. I had run the 10K three times and wanted to explore a route that would take me through more of the city—even if it meant more hills and distance. I was eager to train for both half marathons, viewing them as new experiences and adventures.

Jeff sent me a picture from 2017, taken at the JCC while I was stretching with a TRX. I looked confident, with strong arms and legs—focused and in the moment. I looked… gulp… athletic. But despite my 'seasoned' appearance, I struggled with lunges and wasn't very adept with the TRX.

I reflected on who I was then compared to who I was in October 2022. Was I as focused and oblivious to the camera then? I could have compared numbers on the scale or measurements, but I chose to look deeper. I realized I was still that athletic, focused woman in the fitted top—and I was even more athletic, focused, and strong now, even if I didn't fit into that top anymore.

I had run more races and accomplished things beyond my wildest dreams—two Spartan races, an indoor triathlon, running along challenging trails despite my fear of heights, and racing alone. I was no longer afraid to embrace new challenges Jeff presented. I was more open and brave than I had been in 2017.

Looking at that picture again, I didn't cringe at not fitting into that top or at my weight. The 2022 version of me could do weighted lunges and owned a TRX mounted to the ceiling of my basement gym. Who would have guessed?

Speaking of my basement gym, I continued adding more equipment to my playroom. The open space that once served as a big playroom for my kids had transformed into my own workout area after I became an empty nester! I had kettlebells in various sizes with a stand, along with two stands for my assortment of dumbbells. My gym became a place where I could relax on my yoga mat and strengthen my body with weights. It was where I could get aerobic with my new battle ropes, slam balls, and jump across my Bosu trainer.

I quit Weight Watchers in April, feeling a mix of relief and trepidation, but I truly believed it was the right decision. I hoped someone from WW would reach out to try to win me back. I wasn't sure if I would regret my choice, but after several months, I felt increasingly confident I had done the right thing. I had been a member since June 1986—meaning 36 of my 54 years had been spent as a Weight Watcher. I canceled my membership because I realized I had become a victim of the scale, consumed by anxiety and panic over the number it displayed. Whether at home, the doctor's office, or a WW meeting, I allowed that number to dictate my sense of worth.

My life didn't end when I hit send on my cancellation. Life continued for WW and for me. Despite not loving the numbers I saw, I began to weigh myself with indifference. I stopped the mental games of justifying my diet based on the scale and felt more in control. I knew I was making healthy choices in my eating and workouts.

I continued to work on my mental mindset just as much as my physical self. I would never say no to anything Jeff instructed me to do during a workout (not that he would have let me), but there were plenty of times I questioned if I could actually do it. At the end of one virtual training session, he told me to plank for two minutes. I had done my fair share of two-minute planks, but I still felt panic at the thought of doing it after an intense workout. He told me I could do it—either a straight-arm plank or on my elbows —but I had to hold it for the full two minutes.

Jeff assured me it was all mental and directed me to get in position. Occasionally, he reminded me how much time had passed, but I focused on how much time was left. "It's all mental," he reminded me again. He coached me through, referencing my strength from the Spartan races. I heard him, but I concentrated on holding my plank without dropping my hips or succumbing to the shakiness in my arms.

At one minute and two seconds, he reminded me of the time, and I debated switching to my elbows, but I wanted to maintain my position as long as possible. At one minute and thirty seconds, Jeff said, "You can do this," and in that moment, I told myself I could. I focused on the squiggly designs on the carpet, ignored the ache in my neck, and held my form for the final 20 seconds. 3-2-1. I was done and fell into child's pose. I hadn't let my mental demons convince me I couldn't complete the two minutes. It had been a battle of wills, and I had won!

Another Wednesday, another trail run with Jeff during the few weeks back from Israel. He texted me the address for our run, and as I drove to Adam's Run, I recognized the parking lot and roads leading from the highway. While waiting for Jeff, I stopped at the kiosk and noted the trail map, which labeled the route as 'difficult.' That didn't deter me, nor did the description of a major hill climb. I was ready for this!

As we began our run, turning right onto the trails and tackling a steep hill, I realized we had done this run before. I remembered walking the hills the last time, finding them intimidating. This time, I was determined to approach each hill, trotting or running in place until I reached the top. Jeff led at first—sometimes I was right behind him, other times further back—but all I had to do was follow the trail at my own pace.

I occasionally took the lead while he stopped to take pictures of the beautiful landscape, waterfalls, and undoubtedly a shot or two of me running. I tracked our run on my watch but hardly looked at the time or pace, as I needed to navigate the sticks on the ground and streams to jump across. I felt alive running through Adam's Run, relishing the experience and not worrying about keeping up with Jeff. Although I breathed hard at times, I ran with intensity and a rush I hadn't felt in a long time.

Strava indicated this run was more challenging than my usual efforts—and indeed it was—but it was also an opportunity to revisit a run that had once seemed so hard but was much easier the second time around.

"Tomorrow's run will be tough. It might be the hardest you've ever done."

Those were Jeff's exact words as I prepared for another Wednesday trail run.

Did I freak out? No.

Did I come up with an excuse to cancel? Also no.

I showed up at our meeting point at Columbia Hills, having done everything along the drive *except* think about how difficult that run would be.

I had tackled many hard challenges over the past several years—taking up running, trail running, Spartan races, running in pouring rain, and even in 90-degree heat. I knew there would be plenty of hills and stairs on this run, but I really tried not to dwell on it in those final moments before we started. All I knew was that it would be about five miles—and hard.

We crossed the street by the parking lot and ran up the first steep hill. After reaching the top, we headed down a long series of steps to more trails that led to another road. Jeff mentioned that we had hit a mile, and I cringed, realizing how long it had taken to get to that point. That meant we had another four miles left.

I had already started feeling a twinge in my left calf as we continued onto the Buckeye Trail and did more hill climbing, with some flat sections mixed in to keep things steady. The twinge soon turned into real pain, which I acknowledged out loud. Jeff told me to focus and not let it get to me.

I did my best to run as much as I could... I really did—and I only switched to walking briefly when I felt I had to. We reached a riverbank and turned around, and the run back to the starting point seemed easier and faster. Or should I say... less hard?

When we got to the bottom of the trail and reached the street across from the parking lot, I just ran, heading toward my car as I always did at the end of our runs. Calf pain aside, I needed to finish this very hard run with all the intensity I could muster.

I let myself recover from that tough run—but apparently, not enough. It was now Sunday, and the run had been the previous Wednesday, so I thought that was plenty of time to get back on the treadmill, right?! Wrong! I felt perfectly fine at two miles in and wasn't quite sure what possessed me to think I could run a few additional miles.

My left calf started hurting, and after pushing through, I called it quits at 2.4 miles. After checking in with Jeff about what went wrong, I realized that:

a) I probably should have waited a full week after the trail run before running again, and

b) I should have stopped at two miles when I felt fine.

Lesson learned… well, not quite. I returned to Israel a few days later and allowed my body a day to heal from the flight. I had a good workout on the elliptical the next day—with no pain in my calf. The following day, I thought I was ready for a two-mile easy run outside. I had a guided run podcast to keep me motivated.

I felt a slight tug in my calf at the start but shrugged it off since it didn't make me feel like I had to stop. I saw that I had run half a mile on my watch and thought, "This feels good!" I continued for another .15 mile, and then... that tug turned into a sharp pain in my calf. I tried to slow down and go a little further, but after 30 seconds of easing up, I realized it wasn't going to get any better.

I stopped my watch, feeling frustrated and disappointed. The sharp pain eased a bit and turned into more of a tugging sensation as I walked back to our apartment. I berated myself for not doing more—but I obviously hadn't been ready for it today. A part of me wondered why—after eight days—I wasn't able to get back into it, even when I had held back on distance and pace.

I wanted those two miles to work more than I could picture myself doing three or four miles. I hadn't realized how much my body had been taxed by that trail run in Boston Mills, but I was learning things the hard way.

As I shared with Jeff a few days before, I was okay with giving this the proper healing time it needed and listening to my body—not rushing into anything too soon. I wasn't in a competition, nor was I training for a race (though I had been preparing for the Miami half in January).

Running would be there.

I needed to wait—and focus on giving my joints the much-needed rest they deserved.

Running was indeed there when I allowed myself time to heal properly. I realized I had taken things for granted—assuming that when I went out for a walk or run, everything would go perfectly fine. I believed I could do a hard run and not feel any effects in the hours or days afterward. But I hadn't fully understood just how much my body—specifically my lower body—had been affected by the trail run we'd done nearly two weeks earlier.

I certainly hadn't considered that my entire body would need time to fully rest and recover. I wasn't ready when I ran those two miles on the treadmill five days after the trail run. I wasn't ready when I ran again four days after that, thinking it would be fine. The truth was, I had a calf strain—manageable with certain activities like walking and using the elliptical, but definitely not okay with running so soon after.

I had to take time to recover. In the past, being sidelined brought on panic. I'd worry about not being able to run or walk seriously, and what that might mean for my weight-loss efforts. I didn't know if it was a matter of being older and wiser or simply understanding that this was a blip—not something that needed to spiral into a real setback. Recovery required time.

This wasn't a major injury. It wasn't like when I broke my foot and couldn't bear weight for six weeks. This calf strain was a message: I had done something really hard, and now I needed to learn how to manage things afterward. That meant taking days—or even a week or two—off to get back to a point where I could do something hard again without injury.

When I finally ran on the treadmill and felt no pain, I realized how precious it was to walk pain-free. Each tug-free step reminded me that I'd made the right choice in giving myself the time to rest. I was genuinely grateful for that recovery period. I had stayed active (minus the running), but scaled things back to allow healing. I took walks that were more like strolls, without obsessing over how many calories I was burning or how far I went.

Time did its job. I was back to running—with a deeper appreciation for what my body could do. I learned the hard way that rushing would only backfire. The more I pushed, the more consequences I'd face. I didn't want to pay that price again.

When I finally completed a three-and-a-half-mile run on the treadmill in mid-December, I was elated. It was a distance I had often considered my norm—but this time, it brought me a renewed awareness and appreciation for my ability to run.

After much consideration, I decided to sign up for the Jerusalem Marathon 5K. I had initially wanted to run the half marathon and cover a longer course than the 10K I'd completed three times before, but I realized I just didn't have it in me to train for another half—especially one scheduled only six weeks after the Miami half.

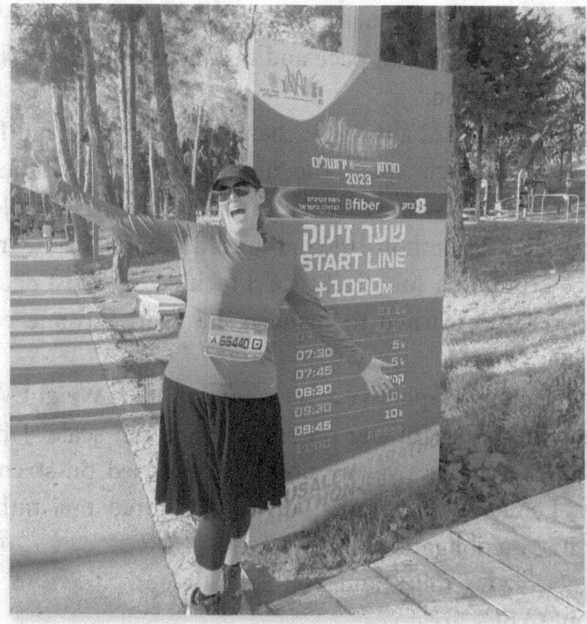

© 2023 Gary Weiss

My boys had nudged me to go for the half, but I knew I wouldn't handle the hilly course well and needed to focus on getting back into running. I didn't want to walk the Jerusalem half, knowing I wouldn't be able to run the entire course. So, I opted for the 5K instead. My husband had walked it many times and assured me it was a flat and enjoyable course.

Though it was a bit late in the game, I officially started training for the Miami half in late December, using run/walk intervals. My brother had suffered an overuse injury during training, and we agreed that if we did any running, it would include walk breaks. We weren't racing this half—we were simply looking forward to completing it together as siblings.

I spent several weeks raising funds for Chai Lifeline, a wonderful organization that supports children and families facing illness and crisis. Jeff developed a great training plan for me—different from those I'd followed in the past. It had a shorter timeline for race preparation since I started later, and it called for increasing my long run by one mile each week during my run/walk intervals to build endurance for the race. On my other running days, I had flexibility with pace and distance, as long as I kept it to 2–3 miles per session.

I didn't finish 2022 any faster than the year before, but I learned not to care so much about the numbers. I ran my fourth half marathon—despite vowing never to do another. I completed my third Jerusalem Marathon 10K in the cold rain and came in second in my age group at a solo trail race. I tackled my most challenging trail run yet and learned to manage the heat, extreme cold, and rain.

I canceled my 30-plus-year membership with Weight Watchers and gradually let go of my obsession with the scale. I began to appreciate the changes in my body as I focused on strength and mobility. I embraced running for all it offered me, rather than viewing it as an obligation.

I logged 431.5 miles and 268 activities on Strava in 2022. It turned out to be a great year.

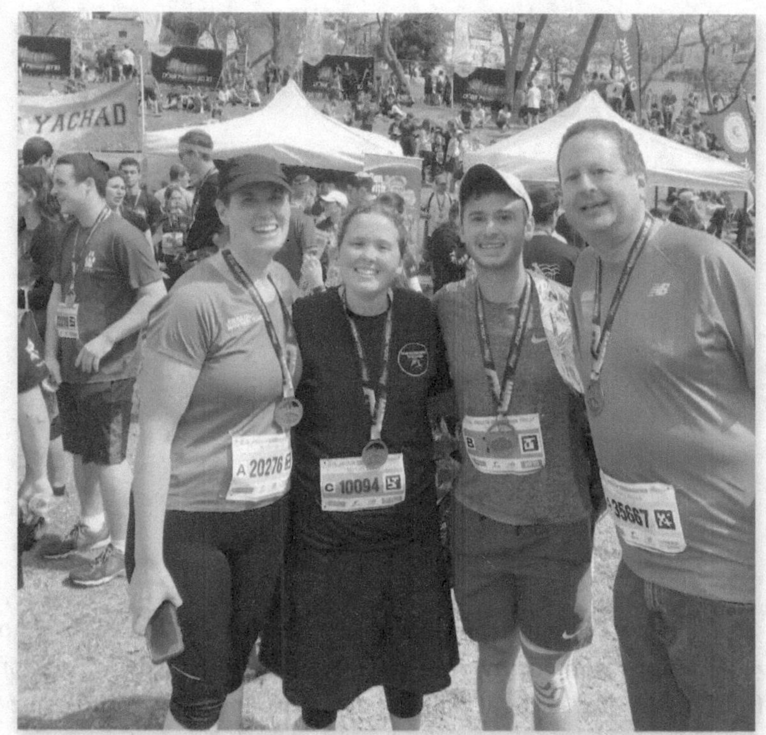

© 2018 Zev Weiss

CHAPTER 9

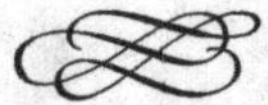

LETTING GO, LACING UP

2023 was about achieving goals and chasing that high. I no longer wanted my runs or races to be defined by pace or finish time—it was about pouring my effort and energy into something and feeling invigorated when I finished. I craved the feeling of strength and invincibility.

I had spent too much time looking back at my running history, wishing I could match my previous paces and times. Deep down, I knew I wasn't the same runner I had been when I first started, but I couldn't help feeling wistful and disappointed in myself. I had focused too much on my lighter weight back then, believing I was fitter simply because I could hit those times.

It took time—and some powerful life coaching from Jeff—to realize that while I was in a different shape at 54 than I was in my late 40s, I was in *better* shape. The 2016 version of me wasn't tackling steep hills on trail runs like the 2023 version. In fact, the 2016 me avoided inclines out of fear—while today's me had completed two Spartan races.

2023 was about achieving goals and chasing that high. I no longer wanted my runs or races to be defined by pace or finish time—it was about pouring my effort and energy into something and feeling invigorated when I finished. I craved the feeling of strength and invincibility.

I had spent too much time looking back at my running history, wishing I could match my previous paces and times. Deep down, I knew I wasn't the same runner I had been when I first started, but I couldn't help feeling wistful and disappointed in myself. I had focused too much on my lighter weight back then, believing I was fitter simply because I could hit those times.

It took time—and some powerful life coaching from Jeff—to realize that while I was in a different shape at 54 than I was in my late 40s, I was in *better* shape. The 2016 version of me wasn't tackling steep hills on trail runs like the 2023 version. In fact, the 2016 me avoided inclines out of fear—while today's me had completed two Spartan races.

I was nine days away from the Miami Half Marathon, feeling all kinds of emotions—but worry and anxiety weren't among them. I approached this "race" with the intention of experiencing it, however my brother and I chose to participate. I felt a peace I'd never known before any past race. There was no pressure about achieving a certain time or viewing it as a competition. I looked forward to the half marathon—enjoying my brother's company and the energy he had described from his experiences as a walker and wheelchair pusher.

I had committed fully to the training plan Jeff designed for this race, seeing it as an event I *wanted* to do, not something I *had* to do. In previous half marathons, I'd been focused on finish times and the effort it took to reach them. The Miami half was different. It was about doing something for others. I had raised over $5,000 for Chai Lifeline and brought awareness to an organization doing incredible work for children and families in crisis.

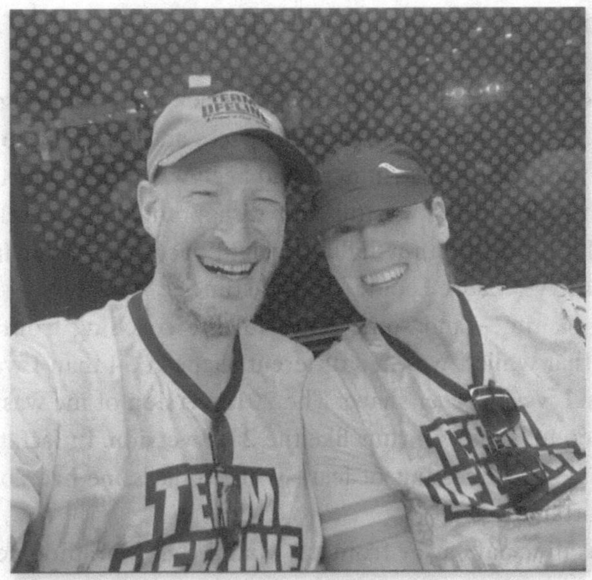

© 2023 Emma Zwick

This was an opportunity I needed more than it needed me. I felt fortunate to be running on behalf of so many who couldn't. I was blessed to be the 54-year-old version of me—not the 46-year-old who was faster and ran more miles. This half marathon was a privilege I no longer took for granted. It was a gift I hadn't always recognized or appreciated, and I was ready to embrace it fully.

My "why" for this race was crystal clear: I was running for something far beyond myself or a medal. I thought about how cancer had touched my life—my maternal grandmother, who lost her battle with breast cancer at 60; her two younger sisters who also faced breast cancer; my paternal grandmother, who passed from lung cancer. I was running for them. For classmates and friends lost too soon. For those who fought and survived.

I was running, grateful that my own breast cancer scares had remained just that—scares. I was running, remembering the fear I felt when our pediatrician sent my now 26-year-old daughter to the pediatric cancer center to test for leukemia—and the relief when she was okay. I was running for my niece, diagnosed at age two with a rare blood disorder, who would be volunteering for Chai Lifeline during race weekend.

I was running for the children and families of Chai Lifeline—the true heroes. And I knew that if I reached a moment in the race where I felt tired or stuck, I would picture the smiling faces from my fundraising page and push ahead to the finish, remembering exactly why I was doing this.

I crossed the finish line of the Miami Half Marathon holding my brother's hand, overwhelmed with emotion but at a loss for words. I got teary, thinking about how this was my last half marathon—and how it had turned out to be such an amazing experience. I hadn't slept the night before, alone in a hotel room and anxious about whether I'd hear my 3:20 AM alarm. But the lack of sleep didn't matter. I was running on pure adrenaline, excited to take part in this race through the streets of Miami.

We boarded a bus at 4:00 AM from our hotel to the starting line. We almost missed our corral because the Miami streets were so congested, and our bus driver was reluctant to let us off where we could easily walk. Micha and I arrived just in time for me to worry about squeezing in a quick bathroom stop—but I decided it was just nerves, and I had already gone plenty of times at the hotel. We were near the back of the corrals but enjoyed watching the earlier waves take off, soaking in the energy. When it was our turn, Micha and I snapped a few selfies and crossed the starting line together.

We ran the first two miles, took a quick bathroom break, walked for about a third of a mile, then returned to running. For the next few miles, we alternated between running and walking as needed. I felt *present* the entire time—thanking police officers directing traffic, cheering on fellow team runners in yellow shirts (even though I didn't know their names), and laughing at the creative spectator signs. I refused to dwell on the discomfort in my glutes and feet and instead reminded myself how lucky I was to be participating in this race.

When the breeze cut through the 74-degree heat, I made a point to feel grateful for it. At mile 6, someone on a loudspeaker shouted, "Who can do a push-up?" And because this race was about the experience, I yelled back, "Me!" I walked over to the mat set up at the side of the road, did one push-up—and then four more because I wasn't satisfied with the first. I smiled. I never would've done that during a race or in public before, but this one was about letting go and letting things happen naturally.

Later, in the second half of the race, I pushed a young woman in a wheelchair for a short stretch and cheered alongside another young woman racing with us. As Micha and I turned onto the final stretch toward the finish line, emotion welled up again. I felt euphoric and exhausted. I felt sad knowing this would be my fifth and final half marathon, having realized I didn't enjoy the training that came with it. But more than anything, I felt blessed, sore, and deeply grateful as we crossed the finish line in 3:00:43—without a care for the clock. (Okay…my Strava said 2:58:15, but that didn't include our bathroom stop after mile 2 when I paused the timer.)

I took a week off afterward—walking on my usual running days and doing light strength work on my moderate to heavier training days. I felt great the next morning and told Jeff, but he advised me to stick to walking no matter how good I felt. It was hard to limit my activity, but I respected and appreciated the recovery process. No matter how "fine" I felt, I knew my body needed time to heal from the half. And because this was a mind/body/spirit journey, I also needed time to mentally and emotionally process what the race had meant to me.

Time would heal, and when I returned to running, I'd be ready.

I was ready. When I ran on February 6, I focused on preparing for the Jerusalem Marathon 5K. My pace ranged between 10 and 11 minutes per mile, but I had initially set a goal to PR this 5K. Achieving that meant putting in serious effort to increase my pace —something I hadn't focused on since the previous winter when I trained for the Jerusalem Marathon 10K. I returned to mile repeats and speed interval runs, hitting fast, unfamiliar numbers on the treadmill. While visiting close friends in Florida, I even managed an easy outdoor run through their neighborhood—navigating the streets without getting lost!

It didn't take long, though, for me to realize I no longer wanted to set records. At first, I was "all in," determined to race it

—but soon, I realized I just wanted to *run* the 5K, not race it. I wanted to stand at the starting line with everyone else, soak up the energy, and take in everything this unique course had to offer. My racing days were behind me—but my running days were far from over.

I still wanted to sign up for races that excited me and enjoy them without obsessing over numbers. I wasn't the runner I had been at 46. Now, I wanted to run for as long as I could—with appreciation and purpose, not with pressure. This shift wasn't about holding myself back—it was about doing what I love, without letting times or paces define the experience. Life was too short not to enjoy every run—whether at a race or on my own.

A few days before the 5K, I compiled a list of my five favorite exercises—and five I'd rather avoid.

Favorites:

1. **Lat Pull-Down Machine** – I loved how my upper body, especially my triceps, felt engaged with each pull.
2. **Chest Presses** – Great upper body work, whether using two 8-pound dumbbells or pushing up with 15s.
3. **Leg Extension Machine** – Burned so good, whether lifting heavy for fewer reps or going lighter with more reps.
4. **Child's Pose** – My go-to cooldown move. I always took a few extra breaths here to center myself after a workout.
5. **Squats** – Whether using the TRX, holding a kettlebell, or doing air squats, this move built strength and made me feel powerful.

Exercises I'd rather skip:

6. **Planks** – I know they're great for the core, but I've never enjoyed holding one—whether for 30 seconds or two minutes.
7. **Row-Ups** – I can do a few with good form, but then I lose it and end up rushing through the rest.

8. **Burpees** – I never know when to jump out of them, and holding proper form in the plank is hit or miss.
9. **Getups** – I've improved, and they're not as dreadful as they once were, but I still forget to reach my hand straight up.
10. **Side Planks** – It always feels like it takes longer to get into position than to hold it.

I couldn't do *any* of these exercises—favorites or not—when I first started working out with Jeff in 2014. But I could do them now, at 54.

The day before the 5K, I slipped on the cobblestone streets of downtown Jerusalem. I was rushing to pick something up for my dad, distracted by thoughts of the race and prepping for a house full of company. The ground had been slick from several days of rain—but whether it was the wet surface, my scattered focus, or just bad luck, I'll never know for sure. I fell hard on my left side. A woman nearby offered to help me up, but I insisted I was fine. I dusted myself off, wobbled through the rest of my errands, and met Gary, who was waiting in the car. I told him I'd taken a spill on Ben Yehuda Street. He gave me that familiar look—equal parts concern and "here we go again."

Ironically, the more active I've become over the years, the more coordinated and flexible I've grown—yet I still manage to fall once or twice a year. I can nail a reverse lunge, yet I'll walk through an empty room and leave with a mysterious bruise on my shin or elbow. This time, I was left with a sore left hip and a big bruise on my right thigh—my latest badge of honor from training.

The next day, I ran the Jerusalem Marathon 5K.

I crossed the start line without expectations—just a desire to run by feel. I began with my friend Tami, who was doing run/walk intervals: a few minutes at a 12-minute-mile pace, followed by short walking breaks. Once we made our way through the crowd of 5K runners and hit the road around the Hebrew University campus, we naturally drifted apart. At the 1K mark, I picked up my pace. Despite the bruises from my fall, I felt surprisingly good. I figured I'd walk or slow down if I felt any pain—but it never came.

Gary had promised me a flat course, but the route had changed, and there were more hills than expected. I tackled them steadily, keeping my breath under control, and focused on enjoying the experience. I never looked at my time—I just ran. And when I reached the finish line, I felt strong, proud, and completely in the moment. It was a great race with a fantastic energy, and I was genuinely glad I had done it.

With the 5K behind me, I gave myself the freedom to run without a training plan or rigid schedule. I was back in control—running three to four days a week, three to four miles at a time. I kept the intensity moderate; anything beyond three miles still felt like I was pushing it. I stuck to my twice-weekly strength sessions with Jeff and followed the Sunday workouts he had built for me. Saturdays became my rest days. I felt good—about where I was and, more importantly, where I was going.

One day in early April, I reflected on what the word *strength* meant to me. My initial thoughts centered around physical strength—holding a squat for 30 seconds, planking for two minutes, chest pressing 30 pounds, and swinging a 25-pound kettlebell. But then I thought deeper about what *strength* truly meant to me.

It was wearing a tank top and capris at the gym after years of hiding in oversized tops and baggy pants. It was getting back up to finish a trail run with blood trickling down my leg after tripping on a step. I realized I had built strength over the years—not just the kind that shows up in muscle tone or biceps, though those were nice too. Real strength came from the decisions I made every day. It was about prioritizing myself—physically and emotionally. It meant facing life-changing health news, caring for one generation while supporting another, and still showing up for myself.

After a week-and-a-half vacation in Orlando for Passover, I saw a number on the scale I didn't like. I knew the scale wasn't the only measure of progress, but I felt the effects of the extra weight—bloating and puffiness. I knew I had to make changes, especially given my current lifestyle: traveling back and forth to Israel nearly every other month, not sleeping well, and having less control over my food choices than I used to.

It was time to get serious.

I began focusing on my water intake, making sure to drink at least 64 ounces a day until it became a habit. That felt manageable, especially compared to trying to limit meals out in Israel. But it was necessary. Eating out was not only expensive, but also "costly" in terms of excess sodium and ingredients that weren't as healthy as they seemed. Improving my sleep was another challenge, but most nights I fell asleep easily and averaged seven hours.

In the nine years I had worked with Jeff, he had me take on various challenges to complement our workouts, my running, and cross-training. There had been a get-up challenge, a modified burpee challenge, and a 30-day burpee challenge I completed a few months later. I had also tackled push-up and squat challenges. I approached each one with a positive attitude (well, maybe not the burpee challenge!) because the moves were specific and planned. When Jeff did the same challenges alongside me, it motivated me—I had support and accountability.

In the third week of April, I began a 90-day core move challenge. Jeff agreed to join me, though we'd each do our own routines and check in daily. This challenge was mine to lead: I needed to come up with a different core move each day and complete 50 repetitions. Jeff advised me not to plan everything out on a calendar, which was my usual tendency. Instead, I'd decide on the move day by day. On heavier leg days, I'd likely avoid lower-body moves like thrusters.

I accepted the challenge with a mix of trepidation and excitement—it was unlike anything I had done before. Creating the list wasn't easy. I initially compiled core-related moves: push-ups, sit-ups, straight-arm planks—50 of each. Then I expanded my list to include exercises using equipment from my basement gym, like the medicine ball and stability ball. Once I thought I'd exhausted my ideas, I turned to YouTube for additional workouts and specific moves.

With 90 moves on my list, I excitedly emailed Jeff and awaited his response. But his feedback wasn't quite what I expected. He told me it was a good start, but many of the moves I had listed weren't truly core-focused—they involved other muscle groups. So, I dug deeper and came up with more targeted core exercises, returning to YouTube for more inspiration. Before I knew it, I had well over 90 moves and felt more confident about the challenge ahead.

Still, I made some mistakes early on. In the first week or two, I attempted more advanced moves. On Day 4, I tried 50 reps of a dumbbell half-kneeling wood chop—25 on each side—a move I'd found in my research. It seemed manageable at first. I started with a 6-kilogram dumbbell, but after a few reps, I realized it was too heavy and switched to a 5-kilogram weight. I finished the set, but my abdominal area started to feel twingey.

The next day was a virtual training session, and I told Jeff about the pain before we began. He had me demonstrate the move over FaceTime. After watching for a moment, he calmly gave me a talking-to. He explained that 12 to 15 pounds was far too heavy for a wood chop—especially a move I had never attempted in our nine years of working together. He emphasized that it wasn't something I should've tried on Day 4 of a 90-day challenge—or even on Day 89!

Fortunately, the abdominal pain disappeared within a day or two, and I continued with the challenge, staying mindful of how I felt during each move. I stuck to exercises I knew I could handle—vertical crunches, sit-ups, standing crunches, and thrusters.

I'd had my share of injuries over the years, whether from falls or overuse. Achilles tendinitis had become a recurring issue, and I had learned the hard way that I needed to stretch both before and after runs—and allow for adequate recovery time after big trail runs or races.

While in Israel, during the 90-day core challenge, I was running on a treadmill one Sunday morning when I suddenly felt a sharp pain in my left foot, right between my ankles. Knowing better than to push through, I immediately stopped the machine and spent the rest of the day icing, elevating, and resting my foot.

The next day, my foot felt a bit better, so I opted for the elliptical—since that movement didn't seem to aggravate the pain. Walking felt okay, but going up and down the stairs in our apartment was painful. I visited a nearby podiatrist who had come highly recommended. After running me through a series of tests I didn't fully understand, he diagnosed me with Achilles tendinitis.

He advised me to focus on upper-body workouts for the next few weeks and to avoid walking and running during that time.

I couldn't figure out what had triggered the injury—I hadn't fallen, twisted my ankle, or done anything particularly strenuous during that casual treadmill run. When I discussed it with Jeff, he mentioned that he'd noticed my shoes seemed a bit loose during our runs and suggested I might need a proper fitting for new sneakers.

The next day, I went to a sporting goods store where the manager scanned my feet and pointed out areas that needed more support. He told me, in no uncertain terms, that I had been wearing the wrong shoe size. But thankfully, he had several options for me to try.

I was skeptical—after all, I'd been wearing size 11½ wide shoes for years, and they had always seemed fine. But then he showed me the results on the Brannock device (yes, I had to Google the name of that foot-measuring tool!)—my feet actually measured as a medium width. He brought out a Brooks model I had worn for years, but in a half size smaller and standard width, and wouldn't you know it—the shoes fit perfectly!

As I walked around the store in my new Brooks Adrenalines, I mentally chided myself for wearing the wrong-sized shoes for so long. This injury might have been avoided had I paid closer attention to how my old shoes were fitting. Lesson learned.

I planned to return to running in a few weeks, once I was completely pain-free. I jokingly told a few people that I had lost weight in my feet. Could they have shrunk because I'd been tracking my macros and calories all these years? Was it from all the running? Inquiring minds wanted to know!

Taking time off from running seemed to aid my recovery, but I admit I opted for easier (not easy) movements. While still in Israel, I used the elliptical twice, taking it easy and making sure to do the stretches my doctor recommended. I felt no tugging or pain in my calves or ankles, so I assumed I was healing. I strolled on the treadmill for a mile or two and felt fine. Once home, I took a day off, and the next day I had a virtual workout with Jeff followed by an easy treadmill walk. No pain.

On Friday, I did an elliptical workout—and there it was. The pain returned with a vengeance by lunchtime. I panicked, worried I had messed things up. I retrieved the massage gun from my bedroom closet and used it on my left calf for 10 minutes, hoping it would knead out the knots. It felt better afterward, but I texted Jeff to let him know the pain had worsened. He suggested I take a few days off from both the elliptical and walking to rest and recover.

As boring and challenging as that sounded, I knew I had to follow orders if I wanted to get back into my routine. Resting wasn't something I enjoyed. I liked to move—and after decades of inactivity, I was finally thriving in my workouts. Movement, whether running or training, was both a physical and mental release for me. But I also wanted to keep moving for years to come—running and training without hobbling or pain.

As boring and frustrating as it felt to take time off, this non-movement would allow me to move later. I knew running would be there for me. I knew there would be summer races and Wednesday trail runs with Jeff. I just had to give this recovery the time and patience it deserved.

When I went out for my first run nearly three weeks after being sidelined, I made sure to warm up properly and stretch. I took it nice and easy, fully aware of how I felt. I noticed a slight tugging sensation in my calf, but I didn't freak out since it wasn't painful. I kept the run to two miles, and by the time I finished, the tugging had disappeared.

As spring turned into summer, my running paces varied in the low to high 10-minute range, but I was too busy enjoying how good running felt to care. I had a greater appreciation for being able to move my feet pain-free, feeling grateful that I could run. I stopped worrying about how long it took me to cover a mile—I was just thankful I could run a mile. Whether on the treadmill or outside, I was doing it because I could. I felt good while running and amazing when I finished.

My focus shifted to running as best as I could in my 54-year-old body and appreciating the gift of running. For too long, I had viewed running as a competition, believing the glory came from crossing a finish line. I learned that running wasn't something I had to do; it wasn't always glorious, and it certainly wasn't a contest. Once I let go of the numbers and stopped comparing my 54-year-old self to my 47- or 48-year-old self, I fell in love with running all over again.

I was in Rocky River, doing a practice run with Jeff for an upcoming trail race. I felt a sense of peace and clarity on the drive home. There was a calmness I hadn't felt in days—maybe even a week. I hadn't felt this calm while running through the trails, especially at the start. Initially, I had focused on getting the run done, needing Jeff to remind me more than once to slow my pace and control my breathing. But once we finished and said goodbye, I felt that clarity during the drive home. I felt healed from this run. I didn't want to listen to music or talk on the phone as I usually did to pass the 30-minute drive. Instead, I used that time to reflect on what that run had given me—even if I initially felt I had little to offer the run.

In early June, I had an epiphany—something was holding me back. I wasn't running to my full potential, and this had been the case for quite a while. Although I was putting in effort, the intensity was lacking. I wasn't pushing myself as hard as I could, allowing my mind to win out over matter. I knew I wasn't going to PR a 5K anytime soon, and I was okay with that. I wasn't going to place in the top of my age group, and I was fine with it. I wanted to run however I was capable of running.

But I had been holding myself back mentally, worried about pushing too hard and increasing my heart rate by running faster than I had been. I knew I could do better than my recent performance. I realized I wasn't in training mode, which may have led me to take it too easy—mistaking 'running according to feel' for running too easily. I hadn't lost my passion for running, but I had lost my way. And I needed to find it again.

I felt more on track when I arrived at the Rocky River Nature Center for the Full Moon 2-mile race. Once again, I ran without a buddy, and it turned out to be a great experience. I parked alongside the parkway near the Nature Center and had plenty of time for a few restroom visits. I felt a bit nervous as I waited for the race to start, wanting to give 100% effort. The first quarter-mile was on the road before heading onto the trails, where I encountered several flights of stairs. I didn't manage them as well as I had hoped and ended up walking them with the other racers. Midway through, I struggled with my breathing and took a short break at the lookout point, berating myself for being out of shape. I made it to the top, got back into a run, and headed to the finish line without worrying about my time.

I had become a regular listener of the *Mind Pump* podcast and emailed them for help with my calorie count. For months, I had stuck to a 2,100-calorie limit, keeping carbs under 25%, but my weight hadn't changed. I shared how I ran a few times a week, worked out with a trainer twice a week, and had tried everything from 24-hour fasts to calorie cuts. Imagine my surprise when I received an email from the show's producer saying they would read my letter on a live episode.

I prepared a script for my Zoom call with Sal, Justin, and Adam on June 13 and felt nervous sharing my story. I explained how I had been trying to find the right calorie count for my activity level, detailing my nutrition attempts and various calorie strategies. I shared my exercise routine, noting that I had only started working out in 2014 after being sedentary for decades. They listened and asked about my breaks during training sessions, to which I replied 30–60 seconds. Later, I realized I had inadvertently given the impression that my work with Jeff focused more on circuit/aerobic training, not mentioning that we had been concentrating on strength training recently.

We didn't conclude how many calories I should aim for, but they recommended a specific daily protein intake and emphasized the importance of including protein at each meal to build muscle, feel satisfied, and improve body composition. They suggested I take a break from running and hike or walk instead, believing that running was hindering my progress.

Initially, I was taken aback at the idea of not running in the immediate future. But as I began to realize that I needed to focus more on building strength—and that running might have actually hindered my progress—I made up my mind to take a break. I wanted to get stronger and leaner, and if that meant putting running on hold for a few weeks, I was okay with that. At the end of our call, they gifted me their *Anabolic* program, and I promised to start it right away.

I took a week off from running and walked instead, but I missed it too much to give it up entirely. I decided I was okay with running on non-training days, keeping the runs simple and low-intensity. I wasn't training for any races and no longer felt the urge to run specific distances in set times. Jeff incorporated much of the Anabolic program into our workouts, but we agreed to start the full program later in July. While in Cleveland for a few weeks, I did as many in-person training sessions at his house as possible. Jeff had a variety of equipment in his garage, which made me feel better having him there to spot me. Taking 90–120 second breaks between sets was a significant change, but those breaks flew by as we chatted and prepared for the next set. I found each workout challenging yet doable, and I even felt athletic!

By the end of June, we were back in Israel for about two weeks, and I aimed to do as many outdoor runs as possible. The problem was, temperatures reached the high 70s by 8 AM, so I started waking up around 7 to get my runs in. July 3 was one such morning where running was on my calendar, but my mind and body hadn't received the memo. Simply put, I wasn't feeling that nudge to run. I had my clothes laid out the night before, planned my route, and knew there was no reason not to go outside.

Checking my phone for the weather, I noticed it was #Rally-ForAli day—a hashtag created by friends and fans of Alison Feller, host of the *Ali on the Run* podcast. I had been a regular listener for years and considered myself a virtual friend, having followed her on Instagram and Facebook since discovering her show. Ali had been diagnosed with invasive ductal carcinoma weeks before and was undergoing a double mastectomy that day. There was no way I wasn't going to run.

I quickly dressed and headed out the door. I walked across the street to my usual starting point, put on a guided run podcast, and pressed start. I felt like I was moving swiftly, but I hadn't checked my watch for a few minutes. As I ran, I pictured Ali smiling ear to ear in her Instagram posts. I dedicated my run to her, as many others would that day, and it turned out to be a great run. I didn't know if I was imagining crossing a finish line at a race where Ali was announcing results or if I was releasing energy or stress I didn't know I had. Regardless, I ran and rallied for Ali, sending thoughts and prayers for her successful surgery and recovery.

Exactly a week later, I had the privilege of meeting internationally renowned marathon runner Beatie Deutsch. I've won a few contests in my 54 years, but this was my favorite! Granted, I once won the key to Kin Shriner's heart in a *Tiger Beat*contest (my name even appeared in the magazine), and I also won a bread machine and toaster oven at a Chinese auction. I even earned a pair of socks for coming in second at last year's Classic at Mastick race. But meeting Beatie? That was truly better than all of that.

I had entered an Instagram giveaway offering various prizes and chose a one-on-one session with Beatie. We planned to meet at a café near Sacher Park—where the Jerusalem Marathon is held—and spent over an hour discussing how I got into running, the races I'd done, our shared experiences with overuse injuries, our kids, and how I could tackle the hills at next year's Jerusalem Marathon 10K. She was sweet, approachable, and generous with her time and advice, sharing wise words about the mental approach to challenges.

At one point, Beatie asked if she could feature me on her Instagram page, *Sunday Strong*, and I agreed—though I didn't quite feel worthy. Later, she posted:

> "I got to meet the incredible Hildee Weiss @momoffive68 today, and I loved hearing her story and how running has improved her life. Hildee started running nine years ago at 46, and she is proof that it's never too late to get in shape. I love the way Hildee is always looking for her next challenge and isn't afraid to step out of her comfort zone. She's constantly working on her mental game. Thanks for inspiring all of us that we GET to run and what a gift that is."

When I read that, all I could think was, *Wow. She got me.*

I hadn't been home for more than 48 hours when I participated in the Full Moon 3-mile trail race with my younger son. I'll explain my use of the word *participate* later, but here are the basics: Yonatan was in town for a few days, and when he heard I would be running a trail race one evening, he asked me to sign him up as well. I was thrilled at the prospect of introducing him to trail running!

The race took place at Pine Hollow, along the trails of Cuyahoga Valley National Park, and it was pouring as we drove there. The downpour made it difficult to see the cars ahead, and part of me wanted to turn around and go home. But then the rain eased to a drizzle, and I continued, explaining to Yonatan that trail running is a different kind of running. It was hard to explain exactly what trail running entailed, but I hoped he would soon see why I loved it so much.

We met up with Jeff in the Pine Hollow parking lot (he was doing his own run) and chatted for a few minutes before we all walked down a grassy hill to the starting line. I was a bundle of nerves, reminding myself this wasn't a race—it was an experience to share with my son. The bell rang, and we started running down a hill that led us into the trails.

Yonatan proved to be a natural, easily navigating the terrain while I struggled to keep up. As for that word *"participate"*? I didn't run the entire course and felt sluggish as I alternated between running and walking, especially when I didn't even attempt the hills and stairs along the route. I'd see a hill ahead and something in me said, *you can't do this,* so I walked. I'd reach the top and switch to running, but I felt defeated and weak—as if it reflected poorly on me, instead of just acknowledging how tough the course was.

I felt bad that Yonatan held back on his usual pace to stay with me, but he kept assuring me he was "good," as he often says, and expressed how happy he was to be running together.

Along the way, he commented on the beauty of being in the woods, and I shared that being in nature was what I loved most about trail running. Yonatan was incredibly encouraging, especially during the last mile when I really felt the heat. He kept telling me how close we were to the finish.

When I saw the finish line at the top of the hill we'd first descended, I told myself to *go for it*. I don't know where it came from, but somehow, I ran up that hill and kept going until we crossed the finish line. I was out of breath and a bit disoriented, and I think I waved to Jeff as I kept walking while he tried to congratulate me.

The course had been more challenging than I was used to. It was extremely humid at 6:30 PM, and I hadn't prepared for that—nor for the hills and stairs. That morning, I had read a post on Instagram by Tina Muir, host of the *Running for Real*podcast. In it, she challenged her audience to use their next run as an opportunity to forget the watch and focus on enjoyment.

During the race, I let Yonatan track our run on his watch and tried to view this race as that opportunity. There hadn't been much to *see* along the trails, but it felt peaceful and meaningful. I was running alongside my son—who wanted to do this race with me! I didn't know if he would take up trail running, but hearing him express his appreciation for it made the heat and hills worthwhile.

We finished the race in 39:48.

The next morning, I shared with Jeff at the start of our virtual training session that I felt the race had been grueling. We discussed how I felt bad for not handling the hills and stairs well, and he reminded me that it had been a race in very humid conditions—and truly challenging. Jeff pointed out that I didn't fully realize what I had accomplished with a run like that.

Before we moved on to our training session, he sent me pictures he had taken of me approaching the finish line, which I waited to view until after we finished. I hadn't known he was taking pictures; all I remembered was how physically and emotionally depleted I felt as I neared the finish. I recalled seeing him at the finish line, but I hadn't thought about whether he had taken photos. I hadn't seen any pictures posted on the race website, so I assumed there weren't any—and I was fine with that.

But then Jeff texted me two pictures of me and Yonatan coming up the hill to the finish line. I looked determined, with my face lowered and focused. It was the same look I'd had in past race photos, but I had never thought much about it. In the past, I would have overthought whether I looked too bottom-heavy. I hadn't considered my appearance beyond the physical. What had been going through my head?!

I took another look at Jeff's pictures and realized I didn't look like I was ready to vomit, as I had feared. I didn't appear to have suffered through intense humidity and a challenging course. I looked strong, present, and determined.

Running—or run/walking—this race with my son allowed us to enjoy time together that we rarely have with everyone else around. We were doing something we loved—running—together, and he had a chance to explore trail running while I tackled a tough course. Looking at those pictures Jeff had sent, I recognized they said so much more about me and how far I'd come.

I went for my annual check-up with my FMD vascular specialist in late July. I had several ultrasounds done in the affected areas, and while there was slight progression, she wasn't overly concerned. We discussed my running, and she suggested I limit my distance to a 10K to avoid overdoing it with my heart rate. I was fine with that restriction, having decided I was happy and done with five half marathons and anything beyond 6.2 miles.

I told her I had shifted my focus to strength training and hoped to lift more than the thirty-pound limit from the previous year. I explained that I had been working with my trainer for nine years and that he was always monitoring my form to prevent injury in the already affected neck and abdomen areas. After confirming I had no intention of entering any CrossFit competitions, my doctor agreed to raise my weight limit to 60 pounds. I was thrilled I had advocated for myself and could work with Jeff on building my strength, boosting my metabolism, and getting fit!

I completed the 90-day core challenge on July 14 with no repeated moves and no pre-planned schedule. This challenge taught me that the core has various areas to work on, depending on the exercise. I could do a sit-up one day, a standing oblique crunch the next, and a Get Up another day. I began to notice a difference in how my core looked and felt compared to when I first started the challenge in April.

The challenge pushed me to create about 80% of the moves, relying on only a few shared by Jeff in his reports. I joked earlier in the challenge that I would someday create a workout video featuring the different moves I had done, followed by a worldwide speaking tour and endorsements from Brooks and New Balance.

For the past few years, I had led a busy life, traveling back and forth to Israel and splitting my time between my kids and grandchildren—which, at times, felt overwhelming. I was so busy flying here and there that I hadn't taken the opportunity to appreciate the experiences I was having, with little downtime. I spent a few weeks in Cleveland between trips to Israel, focusing on doctors' appointments and household tasks.

In late July, my husband underwent emergency retinal detachment surgery, requiring four to six weeks of no travel. We were supposed to go out of town in early August for two weddings and then fly to Israel for over two months. Our son and daughter-in-law were expecting their second child in late August, and we had planned to stay through mid-October to celebrate the Jewish holidays with family. I rescheduled my flight to August 13 to be with Gary for two weeks post-surgery and then make it to Israel in time to help our kids with the baby.

I remember talking to Jeff the day of Gary's surgery. He mentioned that my staying home for an extra two weeks was a gift. He said I was always on the go and needed to take that time to step back and just live. I soon realized how right he was! I knew we could travel once Gary got the thumbs up (which would take 10 weeks), but in the meantime, I used that time to do what I wanted without feeling rushed or pressured. One morning, I went for a walk with a good friend and truly enjoyed the time to chat while walking a few miles. That flexibility allowed me to be out as long as I wanted and go as far as I pleased—because I could. I didn't have a specific time or day to go grocery shopping or bake challah for the Sabbath. That time gave me a kind of freedom I wouldn't have had if we'd stuck to our original plan.

During that time, I went on a trail run with Jeff in Peninsula. As Jeff joked, I went down "like a dollop of whipped cream." I'm not sure if something was in my way, like a stick or a rock, or if I was just distracted by thoughts of Gary at home—but I lost my footing and fell sideways. The moments of falling were a blur; I can't remember exactly how I landed, but I held my left arm up and hollered, "I'm fine." I had dirt all over my palms from using them to break my fall and landed on my right side, but I didn't stay on the ground for more than a few seconds before getting back up and continuing my run. I didn't even pause the Strava app on my watch!

I needed only a minute or two to gather myself—unlike past falls. I jogged along the path just behind Jeff, not thinking about any potential injuries, except for a splinter I felt in my right palm. When Jeff joked about my falling like a dollop of whipped cream, he explained I used to fall like a sack of potatoes. I hoped he meant that a dollop was something graceful... but hey, he was talking about me, and a dollop was a step up from a sack of potatoes!

With no races on my calendar until March 2024, I found myself back in non-training mode, but I still wanted a routine while in Israel for several weeks. As August turned into September and then October, I dedicated myself to training sessions with Jeff and running three days a week. Jeff coached me on strength and conditioning, utilizing the Mind Pump MAPS Anabolic program I received in June—but we had to wait to start until I was in one place long enough.

Through FaceTime, Jeff guided me through movements, weights, and reps. Over time, I increased the weight to keep each set challenging yet doable. I had needed to work on deadlifts for a long time, and I finally got it right while following Anabolic. I started mastering tricep pressdowns using a resistance band tied to the top of the lat pull machine. Squatting with 35-pound dumbbells in each hand became more challenging as I had to remember to take my time and not rush. The hardest part was the 90-second to two-minute break I had to take between sets. I understood the need for recovery time, but I was always ready to move on after 30–60 seconds.

Training with Jeff taught me to slow down, perfect my form, and prepare for the next phase. Could I increase the weights? Could I do more reps? Could I add new moves to challenge myself? I was open to it all.

While the Jerusalem Marathon was still months away, I wanted to prepare for the 10K. My runs included an easy run, a hill/incline interval run on the treadmill, and a speed interval run. The easy run was just that—running without pace, distance, or time in mind, simply to shake my legs out. The incline and speed interval runs aimed to improve my cardiovascular conditioning for better trail running. I followed an interval plan Jeff set up but could modify it weekly if I wanted to increase speed or duration. I had previously said I wasn't in training—but I really was.

CHAPTER 10

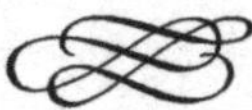

THE NEXT CHAPTER STARTS HERE

Shortly before my 55th birthday, a close friend encouraged me to officially document my fitness journey in writing. I had always thought that sharing posts on Instagram and Facebook was enough—but the idea of compiling my experiences into book format intrigued me. Still, I hesitated. I'd faced challenges publishing my pregnancy loss books and had dealt with untrustworthy publishers and constant rejections. I wasn't sure I wanted to go through that again.

Who would read a book about my journey from inactivity and poor eating habits to becoming an athlete, aside from my closest friends and family? Was there even a market for a story like mine? Did anyone truly care about the ups and downs of my motivation for running?

Well—this is the result of that encouragement. A reflection on the beginnings of my journey and the many runs and races I've experienced along the way. It's been an emotional roller coaster: I've wrestled with motivation, rebuilt my self-confidence, and shifted my mindset. It hasn't been a straightforward path. The earlier years are a bit of a blur, but as I look back at those first runs and recall each race, I see a narrative unfold—a story shaped by every twist, every turn, every detour.

My journey hasn't been easy. I've stumbled many times—literally and figuratively—but I've always managed to get back up. Each obstacle has taught me something new about myself.

Now, as I celebrate turning 55 and more than nine years of embracing fitness, I know there are many more years ahead of me. I want to continue this journey well into my 60s and 70s—and be the woman still participating in 5K races in her 90s, even if it's at a jogging pace. I want to be the grandmother who gets on the floor to play with her grandchildren—and can stand back up, not just watch from the sidelines.

I've come a long way from the 19-year-old girl who preferred taxis over walking five blocks to school. And I know—the best is yet to come!

CHAPTER 11

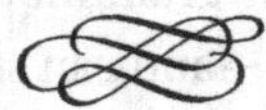

PERMISSION TO REST

I thought I was done sharing my journey, feeling that the fall of 2023 was a good place to end. But I've learned that this journey is never-ending, and I've faced a few more obstacles since then.

I had been dealing with painful degenerative uterine fibroids on and off since November 2021. I managed them as best I could—until they became unmanageable in December 2023. Taking Tylenol every few hours for the pain wasn't helping much, and it began to affect my daily functioning. We had been in Israel for over a month when I felt that familiar pain again. It lasted more than two weeks. I couldn't run or work out, and it impacted my life enough that I consulted my daughter-in-law's gynecologist, who unequivocally stated that I needed a hysterectomy.

Upon returning to Cleveland, I saw my gynecologist, and we agreed that surgery was the only option. I underwent laparoscopic surgery on January 29 and have been recovering at home under many restrictions. I can't lift more than 10 pounds, run for several weeks, or engage in movements involving my abdomen.

When I turned to Dr. Google for information on hysterectomy recovery, I found all the things I couldn't do—but I didn't panic. I didn't worry about gaining weight from not working out for six weeks, and I didn't stress about my inability to run. I accepted my situation, reminding myself that this wouldn't last forever. I had been sidelined before due to injuries and illness. After breaking my foot in 2015, I couldn't run or do any weight-bearing activities for three months—but I returned stronger than ever.

I'm not planning for a personal record at my first race back, but I know that to keep doing what I love for the next 20 or 30 years, I need to accept this moment, give myself grace, be patient, and return with a greater sense of gratitude and appreciation.

And when I do come back, my answer will be:

"What do you want me to do?!"

CHAPTER 12

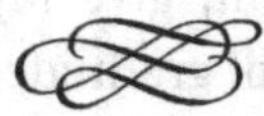

BACK, BETTER, AND BOLDER

This is not the end. In fact, I'm on a new path that began in August 2024, a little over six months after my surgery. I can't pinpoint whether it was the surgery, the slow recovery, or something else entirely, but something shifted during those months when I was in a difficult place. Physically, I felt fully healed within four weeks, yet I followed my doctor's orders and took the full six weeks to ensure I was truly ready.

Mentally, though, it was a different story. As summer flew by and I resumed running and training, something felt off. I started avoiding the NJR running group on Sunday mornings without any real excuse. It wasn't the weather, and I wasn't still sleeping through the 8:15 AM meet-up. Deep down, I questioned whether I could join the group and then run alone, convinced I wouldn't be able to keep up. So instead, I ran solo, gradually working my way back to my usual three- to four-mile runs at a 10:30–11:30 pace. After a few five-mile runs, I only had to stop once in the middle to catch my breath. That was good enough… right? Or so I thought.

In early September, I had a long conversation with Jeff about how I had 'come back' in terms of overall strength and conditioning. I had returned to lifting with increased volume as the summer progressed and was moving with more intensity. Somehow, the conversation turned toward my mental state, and I didn't argue when Jeff said something was missing in me. He noted that I had been at my best when I was regularly doing spin classes and swimming laps as part of my cross-training.

Our session, which usually begins with 15–20 minutes of catching up on personal life and current events, became a therapy session for most of the hour. He asked me what was holding me back, what had diminished my confidence, and when I had lost my joy and drive for running. He pointed out a noticeable dip in my confidence over the past few months—evident when I paused during longer runs to "catch myself." He encouraged me to reconnect with the athlete who once thrived while swimming, spinning, and running with purpose.

I didn't have a clear answer. I had simply stopped swimming and spinning when COVID shut the JCC down—and never returned.

Realizing I wanted to channel that former inner athlete again, I told Jeff I'd dust off my bathing suit and head to the JCC the next morning. Getting back into the pool after so long felt daunting, but once I swam laps for 20 minutes, I realized how much I had missed it—and wondered why I had stayed away for so long. I didn't worry about how I looked in my bathing suit or my lap times. I felt invigorated walking out of the pool and promised myself not to let another four and a half years go by before doing it again.

Jeff led a weekly trail running group that met in places I would have loved to explore, but I always had an excuse not to join. Every Tuesday during our training sessions, I'd ask where the group was meeting that week and how far the run would be—only to come up with a reason not to go. I saw Jeff's pictures and posts from those runs on Facebook and felt a pang of FOMO, yet still avoided the chance to show up.

Finally, at the start of one session, I admitted to Jeff that I didn't think I could keep up with the group and didn't want to hold anyone back. He challenged me to join the next run at Edgewater Park and asked why I was so sure I couldn't keep up. I had no real answer. I asked if there were people in the group who would tolerate my "slower" pace. Jeff shook his head at the word "slower" and assured me I'd have no trouble. As the leader, he had one rule: no runner gets left behind. He promised he'd run with me if I struggled.

So I agreed to go—and I kept my word.

I had never been to Edgewater Park before, but I figured I could handle a three-and-a-half-mile run. After all, I was having one of those "why not?" moments.

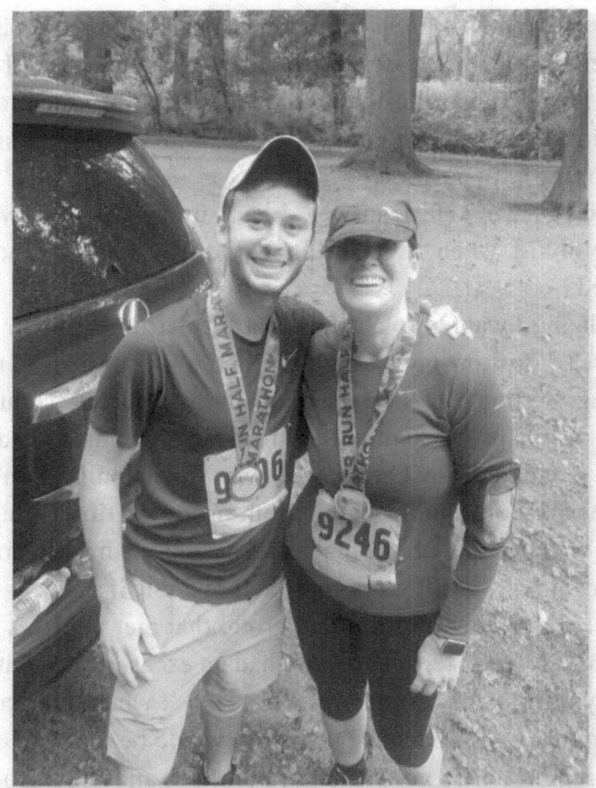

© 2018 Dina Fixler

I showed up the following night and met everyone in the group. They were all friendly, and I felt more at ease as we got started. True to his word, Jeff ran the entire distance with me, while the others were sometimes a bit ahead—and sometimes much farther ahead. But I let go of all my fears and concerns as we ran mile after mile, taking in the beach scenery, the boats at the marina, and the people on the boardwalk. I handled the three-and-a-half-mile run just fine—except around mile two, I noticed we hadn't turned around yet. That "three-and-a-half-mile" run turned out to be 4.7 miles. Not quite the test of endurance I accused Jeff of via text afterward—but definitely a surprise.

As part of rediscovering my inner athlete, I've reintroduced spinning classes into my exercise routine. I hadn't spun since January 13, 2020, but I had truly loved it as part of my cross-training. When COVID hit, the JCC shut down, and my twice-a-week classes came to a halt. But I think there was another reason I stayed away—one I can't quite pinpoint. Maybe I had shifted my focus entirely to running and training with Jeff, which became my core routine. Maybe I was also concerned about the neck movements in spin class and how they might affect my FMD-impacted carotid artery. Honestly, I don't know why I gave it up for so long. But the moment I got back on the bike in Charisse's 9:30 class, I felt like I had come home.

The rush of adrenaline, energy, and excitement reminded me how much I had missed this—my thing.

Since then, I've become a spinner again. I take classes at the JCC when I'm in Cleveland and joined a gym in Jerusalem, where I spin twice a week. I may not be the same spinner I was over seven years ago, but I love it just as much. I've thought about getting a Peloton for home workouts, but there's something about being in a class, moving in sync with the instructor, that really motivates me. For now, I'll keep showing up—and hope that someday, I'll be like the eighty-something woman in my Sunday morning spin class.

I turned 56 on September 30 and took time to reflect on the past year. Traveling back and forth to Israel during a war, undergoing a hysterectomy, and allowing myself the time to heal had made me think I was okay—but that summer, and my conversation with Jeff, revealed otherwise. Running with Jeff's trail group a few times helped me regain the confidence I had started to lose, and once I got back on the spin bike, I felt reconnected to my true self.

I decided to register for the 2025 Jerusalem Marathon 10K and was determined to run the entire course—hills and all—regardless of how long it took. I was eager to sign up and start training. But when I visited the race website, I discovered the race had been postponed to early April... when I wouldn't be in Israel. I was crushed. I had really wanted to run this race, especially after having to skip the 5K I originally signed up for in 2024. I felt mentally prepared to declare my intention and commit to pushing harder over the coming months—with speed intervals, hill work, and mile repeats.

I shared my disappointment with Jeff via text, and he replied, "You can do a 10K in Brecksville that day." My disappointment quickly transformed into determination, and I sent him a 'like' emoji in response. While I wouldn't be running that challenging but beloved 10K in Jerusalem on April 4, 2025, I would still tackle something equally challenging—and equally meaningful—on the other side of the world.

The rest of 2024 had me running with Jeff a few times on the Rocky River trails, braving a bitterly cold Sunday morning with my beloved Aurora running group, and logging many miles on the streets of both Jerusalem and Cleveland. It had been a few years since I'd done a Rocky River workout with Jeff, but we finally made it happen on a wintry November morning. Jeff had been telling me for months that he wanted to make it happen, but he also knew I hadn't been ready. Physically, he believed I could do it. But it had taken time for me to get there mentally—and now, I was.

What *"this"* involved was running in and out of a ladder, jumping rope with free handles, doing squat jumps and holds with a TRX strapped to a tree branch, slamming a weighted ball into the muddy ground, and finishing bicep curls with a resistance band. Then came a second, more challenging interval. Through it all, I did my best not to focus on the people passing by in cars or on foot. I stayed in the moment. I focused. I breathed.

Once the workout wrapped up, Jeff turned to me and said, "Get ready for a nice little two-plus-mile trail run." A few months earlier, I might've told him (and myself) that I was too tired, or that the workout had been hard enough. But not that morning. That morning, I was ready for anything. I was back—physically, mentally, and everything in between.

I finished 2024 with a sense of satisfaction and deep contentment. For the first time in a long while, I was truly happy with myself. It had nothing to do with the number on the scale or the size on a clothing tag. It had everything to do with the shifts I had made in recent months. As I said goodbye to 2024 and stepped into 2025, I found myself running with a heightened sense of awareness and appreciation. I run because I *want* to—not because I have to. I spin because I *love* how I feel pedaling to the beat, riding the rhythm, riding *myself* back to life. The adrenaline rush stays with me for hours.

It feels good to do what I love. And even better to feel good while doing it.

I'm no longer the same wife and mother who first walked into Jeff's office back in 2014, too afraid to say out loud that I wished I could run. I've lived through highs and lows, setbacks and triumphs. I've fallen—physically and metaphorically—but I've always gotten back up. And through it all, I've become stronger, more resilient, and—gulp—a little more confident.

You want me to do what?!

Let's go!

ACKNOWLEDGMENTS

Denny Krahe, thank you for writing the foreword to this book. I asked you because I respect you—as a coach, podcast host, athlete, and all-around great guy. You read my manuscript, and you *got it*.

Jeff, you've been there every step of the way since that fateful day in July 2014. You've been available nearly 24/7 to answer my questions, however trivial. You've taught me so much about fitness and nutrition, and you've also allowed me to take the lead at times—creating my own training plans and guiding our trail runs. You encourage me when I'm feeling down and push me when I think I can't go any further. You're tough on me when I need it and full of praise when I've earned it. You believed in me when I didn't believe in myself, pushing me out of my comfort zone to achieve things I never thought possible. I know it's because you believe I can. You're so much more than a trainer—you're one of my closest friends, and I'm forever grateful for everything you've done and continue to do.

And thank you to Mirvat for all the race photos, being the best stylist, and ensuring the towel didn't drop in the parking lot.

To Denny Krahe, Steve Carmichael, Ali Feller, Carrie Tollefson, Matt Chittim, Martinus Evans, Latoya Shauntay Snell, Lindsey Hein, Jill Angie, Duane Scotti, Dimity McDowell, Sarah Bowen Shea, Jordan Syatt, Jonathan Levitt, and the team at Mind Pump—each of you played a role in my journey through your podcasts. Whether it was your own voice, your guests, or the topics that resonated with me, you helped get me off the couch and prioritize both my physical and mental health.

To my running and walking friends—Caroline, Cheryl, Debbie, Frankie (and Reese's), Kasey, Kimi (and Belle and Bailey), Lisa, Marla, Miki, Tami, Tracy, and all the Sunday Aurora group run ladies and NJR members—our time together on walks and runs has meant the world to me.

Caryn, thank you for suggesting I write about my fitness journey back in September 2023, when I had some free time and a dream that felt unreal. Your support means so much, and I appreciate you being a wonderful friend and partner in crime to our kids and grandsons.

Dina, thank you for meeting me at mile 3 of my first 5K and guiding me to the finish. I'm grateful for our drives to the River Run and Rite Aid races. You have been a dear friend, role model, and inspiration. I wish you many more years of running and racing.

Batsheva, you have always been my cheerleader. Thank you for reading my blogs and encouraging me on this fitness journey.

Bonnie, your enthusiasm for strength training inspired me to lift, tone, and get strong. I can't thank you enough for being both a friend and role model.

To my KC crew, I found you by chance on the WW message boards, and I've developed real friendships with each of you. We've laughed, cried, celebrated, and mourned together. We are a mighty group, and I appreciate your continued support of my journey.

To my parents—thank you for reading my blogs and teaching me to get back up after I fall, no matter how often it happens. You've supported all my running and fitness efforts with pride and disbelief that I'm the same little girl who used to stumble.

To my in-laws—thank you for supporting everything I do and nudging me to prioritize myself. And thank you for giving me Gary!

To my children—Yaffa, Yoni, Seth, Penina, Miriam, Yonatan, Kayla, Liat, and Noah—thank you for encouraging and cheering me on. I wanted to be a better, healthier mother to all of you, and I hope this journey has allowed me to be a role model. Thank you for all the runs and races we've shared—and for the car rides when I needed shelter from the rain.

To my grandchildren—Ezra, Arielle, Aidan, Orli, and Shai—you are one of the main reasons I do all of this. I want to be the kind of grandmother who gets on the floor to play with you, has the energy to dance with you, and can do 'Round the Clock.'

And Gary…

You asked me for a second date, and then another, and despite my complaints about walking all those blocks in Manhattan, you never gave up on me. You've risen at dawn to drive me to races and been there at the finish lines—beaming with pride, encouragement, and a bit of wonder. You are my greatest cheerleader, and I treasure you for all that you are.

I love you more than words can say.

ABOUT THE AUTHOR

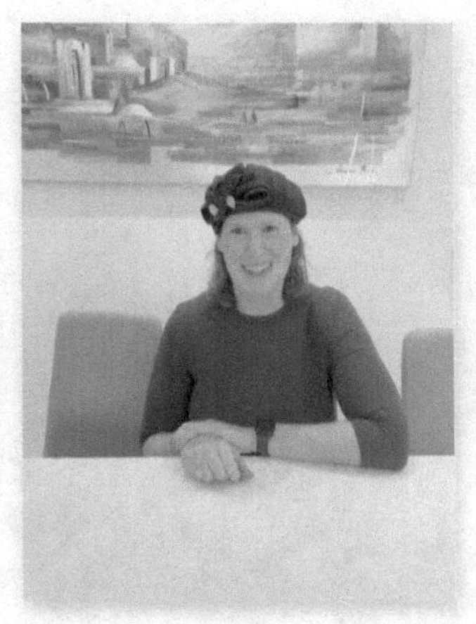

Hildee Weiss is a wife, mother, and grandmother whose work spans topics ranging from soap operas and parenting to pregnancy loss and fitness. She published *Forever Our Angels* and *Remembering Our Angels: Personal Stories of Healing From a Pregnancy Loss* under the pen name Hannah Stone. Hildee contributed a patient's perspective on pregnancy loss to the book *Recurrent Pregnancy Loss,* published by Springer in 2018. She has been a featured guest on the Diz Runs, Run Buzz, and Mind Pump podcasts. Hildee chronicles her running and fitness journey on her blog: youwantmetodowhat.home.blog.

www.ingramcontent.com/pod-product-compliance
Lightning Source LLC
LaVergne TN
LVHW031343150826
845673LV00009B/2843

* 9 7 9 8 8 9 4 4 1 0 3 2 6 *